THE STIGMA OF MENTAL HEALTH IN THE AFRICAN AMERICAN COMMUNITY

Antonio Brigham, MSN-Ed, RN

The Stigma Of Mental Health In The African American Community

All rights reserved. No part of this book may be reproduced in any form or by any electronic or mechanical means, including information storage and retrieval systems, without permission in writing from the author. This book was professionally written, edited, and formatted. It is not a pre-published work and remains the copyrighted property of the author.

This book is written to provide helpful information on the subjects discussed in it. This book is only meant to provide the reader with basic knowledge of certain topics, and it does not guarantee results. This material is for educational and entertainment purposes only. Though the information contained in this book is well thought through and carefully written, the author accepts no responsibility for any errors or omissions that may be made. Additionally, the author accepts no liability by the publisher for any damage, losses, or costs resulting from using this material.

All trademarks and registered trademarks appearing in this book are the property of their respective owners and are used only to describe the products provided directly. Strenuous effort has been made to properly capitalize, punctuate, identify, and attribute trademarks and registers according to industry standards.

ISBN: 978-1-915930-80-4 PAPERBACK
ISBN: 978-1-915930-81-1 HARDBACK
ISBN: 978-1-915930-82-8 EBOOK

Contents

INTRODUCTION 6

01. MENTAL HEALTH STIGMA IN AFRICAN AMERICAN
COMMUNITY 9
The Mask of Strength: How Mental Health Stigma was Born .. 10
Post-Civil War Era and the Rise of Stereotypes 11
Jim Crow Laws and the Effects of Segregation on Mental
Health 12
The Effects of the Tuskegee Syphilis Experiment 13
Media Representations of Mental Illness 14
The Impact of Mental Health Stigma in the African American
Community Today 15

02. UNDERSTANDING TRAUMA IN AFRICAN AMERICAN
COMMUNITY 17
Common Types and Sources of Trauma in African American
Communities 18
The Impact of Trauma on Mental Health 19
Recognizing the Signs of Trauma in Individuals and Families 21
Understanding How Trauma Can Be Passed On
Intergenerationally 22
The Relationship Between Trauma and Substance Abuse ... 23

03. PREVALENCE OF DIFFERENT MENTAL HEALTH
CONDITIONS 26
Common Mental Health Conditions in African American
Communities 27
    Depression 27
    Anxiety 29
    Bipolar Disorder 30
    Schizophrenia 32
    Post-Traumatic Stress Disorder (PTSD) 33
Diagnosing Mental Health Conditions: Challenges and
Solutions 34
Different Types of Therapies 35

04. CULTURAL RESPONSES TO MENTAL HEALTH 37
How Cultural Norms Impact Mental Health Conversations 38
The Role of Religion in Mental Health 40
The Power of Family Dynamics 42

05. ACCESS TO MENTAL HEALTH CARE 46
Economic Challenges and a Lack of Coverage 47
Systemic Discrimination in Health Care Settings 49
Distance From Services and Transportation Issues 50
Language Barriers as an Obstacle 51
Limited Resources in Underserved Communities 53
Unclear Diagnosis and Treatment Plans 54
The Fear of Renewed Discrimination Due to Seeking Help ...55

06. OVERCOMING THE MENTAL HEALTH STIGMA 57
Challenging Popular Misconceptions and Myths 58
Creating a Supportive Environment for Mental Wellbeing ...59
Educating our Communities about Mental Health 61
Seeking Professional Help and Treatment 62
Increase Funds and Resources for Mental Health Services ...64
Working with Community Leaders to Advocate Mental Health ...65
Creating Safeguards Against Discrimination and Racism 67

07. CULTURAL COMPETENCY OF MENTAL HEALTH PROVIDERS 69
The Importance of Understanding the Unique Cultural Experiences 70
Addressing Disparities or Stigmas Associated with Certain Cultures 72
Providing Respectful Care to Diverse Populations 73
Incorporating Cultural Practices into Treatment Plans 74
Developing a Self-Awareness of Own Biases and Strengths ..76

08. STRATEGIES FOR IMPROVING ACCESS TO MENTAL HEALTH CARE 79
Increasing Funding for Mental Health Treatment 80
Improving Transportation Options 81
Reducing Language Barriers 83
Utilizing Technology to Access Mental Healthcare 85

09. EXPLORING SELF-CARE AND COPING MECHANISMS FOR MENTAL HEALTH ISSUES. 87
  Mindfulness Practices 89
  Writing and Journaling 91
  Yoga.. .. .. .93
  Exercise.. .. .. .94
  Dietary Changes.. .. .. .96
  Practicing Self-Compassion 98

10. FAITH-BASED APPROACHES TO MENTAL HEALTH .. .100
  Prayer and Other Religious Practices 101
  Religious Counseling for Mental Health Issues 103
  How Churches Can Play a Part in Improving Access to Care 104
  Overcoming Obstacles in Implementing Faith-Based Practices 106

11. UPLIFTING STORIES OF AFRICAN AMERICAN MENTAL HEALTH ADVOCATES.. .. .. .108
  The Story of Taraji P. Henson. 109
  Charlamagne Tha God 110
  Joy Harden Bradford .. .. .111

12. MOVING FORWARD WITH MENTAL HEALTH CARE IN AFRICAN AMERICAN COMMUNITY . .. .114
  Positive Representation in the Media: A Step in the Right Direction 115
  Accessibility to Quality Care: Creating an Inclusive Environment 116
  Taking Action Together for a Brighter Future 117

CONCLUSION.. 119

GLOSSARY.. .. .. .122

ADDITIONAL RESOURCES. .. .. .127

ACKNOWLEDGMENTS.. .. .. .129

AUTHOR'S NOTE 130

REFERENCES 131

Introduction

This book is an exploration of the complex and often misunderstood issue of mental health in the African American community. While this is a topic that has been discussed for decades, it remains largely ignored in mainstream conversation. This book seeks to bring attention to the prevalence of mental health issues in African American communities and provide readers with the requisite knowledge, understanding, and encouragement about the need to seek help for their mental health struggles.

Mental health is an issue that often goes unaddressed in the African American community due to a variety of reasons, such as shame, fear, and a lack of access to quality mental health care. This book seeks to address these issues head-on and educate readers about their mental health while encouraging them to seek help if needed.

Mental health stigma is one of the biggest barriers to effective mental health care in the African American community. This book will discuss why this stigma exists, how it can be overcome, and provide readers with knowledge and resources for improving their mental health. Additionally, it will highlight stories from those who have experienced the stigma of mental health and show how they have worked through it to get help.

For those who have experienced trauma or struggle with depression or anxiety due to living in an oppressive society—this book is for you. It will provide insight into the history of mental health stigma in African American communities and show how it has been perpetuated through cultural norms and attitudes.

By understanding the history of mental health stigma and how it affects African American communities, readers will gain insight into what needs to be done to create a more inclusive understanding of mental illness. They'll also learn about strategies for overcoming mental health stigma in their own community, such as changing attitudes toward mental illness, educating people about its effects, and providing support networks for those living with a mental health condition.

Mental health in African American communities is like a garden that has been neglected for too long. The soil is dry and lacks the nutrients needed to nurture growth, while weeds of stigma have choked out any prospects of blooming. In order for this garden to thrive, it needs care and attention, which has been all too often lacking.

This book serves as a blueprint for how to start rejuvenating this garden. It will provide readers with insight into what mental health issues look like in African American communities and ways they can begin cultivating their own mental well-being. It also looks at strategies for overcoming mental health stigma and provides information on resources available to those living with mental illness.

The first step in rebuilding this garden is recognizing the symptoms of mental illness and understanding how different conditions are diagnosed and treated. This book examines the types of mental health conditions most commonly seen in African American communities, including depression, anxiety disorders, bipolar disorder, schizophrenia, post-traumatic stress disorder (PTSD), and substance abuse.

Moreover, it looks at cultural norms and societal influences that have impacted attitudes toward mental health in African American communities. Recognizing these influences will help readers understand why seeking help may be difficult for some individuals due to shame or the fear of stigmatization.

In order for this garden to bloom again, it needs more than just knowledge—it needs support and resources in the form of access to quality mental health care. This book discusses ways to increase funding for treatment, improve transportation to healthcare facilities, reduce or eliminate language barriers, increase community awareness about mental illness, and create more culturally-sensitive services tailored to the needs of individuals living with mental health conditions.

Self-care practices and coping strategies are also essential components of this garden. Readers will learn different techniques for managing symptoms and improving their overall well-being, such as mindfulness, journaling, yoga/meditation, support groups, exercise/dietary changes, medication, religious counseling, prayer, and meditation.

Finally, this book encourages readers to look beyond themselves for inspiration when it comes to cultivating their own mental health garden. It includes stories from African American mental health advocates who have overcome their struggles with mental illness and become powerful role models for those in similar situations.

By taking the necessary steps to care for this garden, readers can begin creating a more inclusive understanding of mental health in their own community and make sure everyone has access to quality care and support.

This book is a call to action for all of us to take steps toward creating a more understanding and supportive environment for those living with mental health issues in the African American community. With knowledge, understanding, and resources, we can overcome the stigma that has held back progress for so long.

By joining together and making our voices heard, we can ensure everyone has access to quality care and support. It is entirely our responsibility to create a future where mental health is seen as something beautiful rather than shameful—a future where everyone has access to the help they need. Together, we can make this garden blossom!

CHAPTER ONE

MENTAL HEALTH STIGMA IN AFRICAN AMERICAN COMMUNITY

Mental health awareness has come a long way, but there's still much work to be done. Nowhere is this more evident than within the African American community, where stigma around mental health continues to exist. In this chapter, we'll explore the history of mental health stigma in African American communities and how it has been perpetuated through cultural norms and attitudes. Additionally, the chapter takes a look at the recent dynamics of mental health within these communities.

Change doesn't come easy, but together, we can make sure everyone has access to the help they need without fear or shame. Let's get started!

The Mask of Strength: How Mental Health Stigma was Born

Throughout history, African Americans have been seen as strong and resilient. This societal narrative of strength has served to mask the reality that mental health issues exist within the community. Unfortunately, this belief in "strength" has only perpetuated mental health stigma, making it difficult for individuals in the community to access health care and support or even recognize their own needs.

The roots of mental health stigma in the African American community can be traced to the time of slavery. Slave masters often viewed the enslaved with suspicion and fear, believing that any sign of distress or illness was evidence of weakness and rebelliousness. This manifested itself in harsh treatment as well as a lack of access to medical care. Slaves were expected to be stoic in the face of physical and emotional suffering, which was seen as a sign of strength.

The legacy of slavery has had a lasting impact on how African Americans view mental health issues in recent times. Even though times have changed and people are no longer enslaved, this narrative of "strength" is still pervasive in some sectors of the community. This stigma prevents individuals from seeking out help for mental health issues or even recognizing that they may need it.

The issue of mental health stigma is further complicated by a lack of resources in the African American community. Many African Americans struggle to access quality healthcare due to economic and educational disparities. This can be particularly true for those living in rural areas, where there might not even be a doctor or hospital nearby. As a result, many individuals are unable to receive mental health care or do not know how to find it.

This lack of access to resources is compounded by another factor: fear. In the African American community, there is often a fear of being judged or stigmatized if one were to talk openly about mental health issues or about their status. This fear can partially be attributed to the legacy of involuntary commitment that has plagued African Americans since slavery. To this day, there remains a distrust among African Americans of the healthcare system and its ability to help those in need of care.

Post-Civil War Era and the Rise of Stereotypes

The end of the Civil War marked a new era for African Americans, but unfortunately, it also saw the rise of stereotypes that would perpetuate mental health stigma for years to come. During this period, African Americans were seen as lazy, unintelligent, and prone to emotional outbursts. This led to a belief among some members of society that individuals from the community were inherently weaker than their white counterparts when it came to dealing with mental health issues.

These stereotypes were further perpetuated by the medical profession at large. Physicians often diagnosed members of the African American community with disorders such as "drapetomania," which was supposedly a mental disorder causing slaves to run away. This diagnosis was based on the false assumption that African Americans were unable to control their emotions and behaviors in the same manner as whites.

At the same time, there was also a belief among some members of society that African Americans possessed an innate ability to cope with extreme physical and emotional suffering due to their genetic makeup. This idea of "superhuman resilience" served only to reinforce existing stereotypes and prevent individuals from seeking help for mental health issues.

The combination of these factors created an environment where mental health stigma could thrive. As a result, many African Americans faced significant barriers when it came to accessing care or even recognizing their own needs. This in turn further perpetuated the cycle of stigma, as individuals were likely to hide their mental health struggles out of fear of being judged or labeled as "weak" by members of their community.

Additionally, this environment often discouraged individuals from engaging in self-care activities, such as exercise, meditation, and therapy. This lack of self-care only served to worsen existing mental health symptoms and increase stigma within the community.

Jim Crow Laws and the Effects of Segregation on Mental Health

The era of segregation, known as Jim Crow, has had a profound effect on the mental health of African Americans. The segregation laws created a two-tiered system that denied individuals equal access to resources, education, and employment opportunities as their white counterparts. These laws were inherently discriminatory as they failed to recognize the fact that all human beings are born free and equal in dignity and in rights, irrespective of race, ethnicity, or gender. Consequently, this discriminatory tendency against African Americans further nurtured mental health stigma within the community by forcing people to hide any signs of distress or illness rather than seek care and support.

The effects of Jim Crow laws were compounded by the fact that these obnoxious laws prevented African Americans from receiving the same health care as their white counterparts. Mental health facilities and hospitals typically refused to administer treatment to members of the community, leaving many individuals without access to proper care. This led to an increased sense of isolation among those experiencing mental health issues, which only served to worsen their symptoms.

At the same time, segregation also meant that African Americans had fewer role models in the medical field. This further discouraged individuals from seeking help as they felt there was no one they could turn to—someone who would understand their situation and provide appropriate care.

The legacy of Jim Crow lives on today in many aspects of American society, including healthcare. Studies have shown that African Americans are less likely to receive adequate mental health treatment than whites due to a combination of economic barriers, distrust of the healthcare system, and fear of judgment or rejection from members of their community.

In addition, studies have revealed that African Americans living in areas with high levels of segregation are more likely to experience mental health issues, such as depression and anxiety. This confirms what many in the community already know: segregation has had a devastating effect on mental health and continues to prevent individuals from receiving the care they need.

The Effects of the Tuskegee Syphilis Experiment

The Tuskegee syphilis experiment was a medical study conducted by the U.S. Public Health Service from 1932 to 1972 that sought to examine the impact of syphilis on African Americans. During this time, hundreds of people—who were mostly poor black men—were enrolled in the experiment without their knowledge or consent and denied access to treatment for this highly contagious disease.

This unethical experiment caused deep distrust among many African Americans toward the medical establishment, leading them to avoid seeking care—even when they most needed it—out of fear of mistreatment or exploitation. This mistrust has had a lasting impact on mental health stigma within the community as individuals are less likely to access care out of fear of being judged or mistreated.

The Tuskegee syphilis experiment also serves as a stark reminder that African Americans were, and still are, disproportionately affected by mental health issues due to the legacy of systemic racism. It is not hard to see how the trauma inflicted on these men has been passed down through generations, leading to an increased risk for mental health issues, such as depression and anxiety, among members of their community.

Additionally, the Tuskegee syphilis experiment has had a lasting impact on rates of syphilis among African Americans. The experiment, which lasted for 40 years, saw hundreds of black men enrolled without their knowledge or consent and denied access to treatment. This unethical study caused deep distrust among African Americans toward the medical establishment, leading to an increase in cases of untreated syphilis.

Due to limited access to quality healthcare and the fear of mistreatment or exploitation, many African Americans are reluctant to seek medical care even when it is necessary. As a result, the rates of syphilis have been higher within this community than among other racial groups for decades. A report from the Centers for Disease Control and Prevention (CDC) found that black men were more likely to be diagnosed with primary and secondary syphilis infections—a rate that has been steadily increasing—than white men.

This disparity can partially be attributed to economic disparities as well as structural racism, which limits access to quality healthcare for many African Americans. However, it is also important to recognize the role that mental health stigma plays in this issue. Many individuals are unwilling or unable to seek out care due to fear of judgment from members of their community or rejection from healthcare professionals.

Media Representations of Mental Illness

The media has an important role to play in shaping our perceptions of mental health. Unfortunately, when it comes to African American communities, media reportage often reinforces existing stereotypes and perpetuates stigma.

For example, the majority of television shows featuring African Americans portray them as either criminals or uneducated buffoons who are out of touch with reality. This representation of African Americans reinforces the false idea that mental illness is a sign of weakness and perpetuates the notion that those with mental illness are not capable of leading successful lives.

In addition to this, when mental health issues are addressed in the media, it is often done in a sensationalized or comedic way that trivializes the seriousness of the issue and contributes to misunderstandings and stigma around mental health within African American communities.

By portraying mental health issues as something laughable instead of being taken seriously, people may be less likely to seek help or even discuss their problems openly. Unfortunately, this lack of open discussion and awareness can lead to more serious consequences, such as increased suicide rates in African American communities.

It is therefore important for the media to take responsibility for its role in shaping public perception and start accurately representing mental health issues in African American communities. It is only by doing so that we can begin to reduce stigma and open up conversations about these issues, which are essential steps toward achieving better mental health outcomes for everyone, irrespective of race or ethnicity.

The Impact of Mental Health Stigma in the African American Community Today

The effects of mental health stigma can be far-reaching and have long-term implications for individuals in the African American community. Those suffering from mental health issues may feel isolated due to a lack of understanding from their peers, leading to feelings of shame and guilt. This can lead to an increased risk for depression and anxiety, as well as other mental health disorders, such as posttraumatic stress disorder.

Without proper access to care or even recognition that they may need help, individuals in the African American community are more likely to self-medicate with drugs or alcohol, further exacerbating their condition. Additionally, without treatment, those suffering from mental illnesses are at greater risk for developing more serious medical conditions, such as heart disease or diabetes.

Mental health stigma also has implications beyond the individual level. Empirical studies have shown that its effects can reverberate through entire families and communities due to its influence on communication patterns and relationships. It can also perpetuate existing economic disparities within the African American community by limiting access to resources and preventing individuals from seeking help or even recognizing their own needs.

Finally, mental health stigma also has a social cost associated with it: unfair judgment and discrimination toward members of the African American community who might be struggling with these issues. This can further increase feelings of isolation and make it difficult for those affected to find support from their peers when needed.

Mental health stigma has been a longstanding issue in the African American community, one that is deeply rooted in false stereotypes and misconceptions. By taking the time to understand how mental health stigma affects this community, we can start to have more meaningful conversations about this phenomenon and take steps toward reducing its impact.

It's important for everyone—not just those in the African American community—to learn about mental illness and understand its effects on individuals, families, and communities as a whole. Only by doing so can we hope to break down existing social barriers and create a more open dialogue around these issues. With increased awareness and understanding, we can begin tackling mental health stigma in African American communities head-on and move toward a brighter, more inclusive future for all.

CHAPTER TWO
UNDERSTANDING TRAUMA IN AFRICAN AMERICAN COMMUNITY

African American communities have long battled the effects of trauma. While it may not always be visible on the surface, this trauma can manifest in a variety of ways and create a ripple effect throughout families and communities. This chapter dives into exploring what trauma looks like in African American communities and its impact on mental health.

We'll take a look at some of the common types and sources of trauma, as well as how to recognize its effects on individuals and families. With this knowledge, we can create better strategies for providing assistance and support to those in need. So let's jump right in!

Common Types and Sources of Trauma in African American Communities

Trauma can be defined as any experience that causes physical or emotional pain, suffering, and distress. It is a normal response to an abnormal event, like a natural disaster or violent act, and it can also be caused by ongoing adverse life experiences, such as poverty, discrimination, and oppression.

In the African American community, trauma has a long and complicated history. The legacy of slavery, segregation, and structural racism has created an environment where Black people are more susceptible to traumatic experiences. This is further compounded by the fact that African Americans often experience higher rates of poverty, violence, discrimination, and other forms of social injustice than their white counterparts.

There are several different types of trauma that can affect individuals and communities in different ways. These can include physical trauma due to life-threatening events, such as accidents or natural disasters; psychological trauma caused by ongoing stressors, such as racism or poverty; post-traumatic stress disorder (PTSD) caused by single traumas, such as war or sexual assault; as well as developmental trauma experienced during childhood due to neglectful parenting or other adverse childhood experiences.

One of the most common sources of trauma experienced by African American communities is the legacy of slavery, discrimination, and segregation. This includes the physical, psychological, and economic effects that stem from this history. For example, African Americans are more likely to experience poverty due to disparities in income and employment opportunities which can lead to higher rates of crime and violence in their communities. Additionally, they may endure racial slurs or other forms of discrimination based on their race or ethnicity.

Another source of trauma for African American communities is police brutality. This type of trauma often occurs when law enforcement officers use excessive force against individuals or racial profiling when making arrests, which can have long-lasting effects on a person's mental health. Furthermore, there are ongoing reports of police officers failing to de-escalate tensions in African American communities which can lead to further trauma.

Violence is another source of trauma experienced by African American communities. This type of trauma can include physical or emotional abuse, sexual assault, and homicide. It often results in an individual feeling unsafe and helpless, leading to long-term mental health issues, such as post-traumatic stress disorder (PTSD).

Finally, poverty is a major source of trauma for African American communities. The effects of poverty can be particularly detrimental due to disparity in remuneration and the limited access to resources and opportunities available in low-income neighborhoods or areas that are largely populated by people of color. This lack of resources can lead to higher rates of crime and violence as well as mental health issues, such as depression and anxiety.

The Impact of Trauma on Mental Health

It is an undeniable fact that trauma has a profound impact on the mental health of African Americans, which can manifest in many ways. Trauma does not just affect individuals but also entire communities that have been exposed to various forms of violence and oppression. Understanding the full scope of this impact is essential to developing effective strategies for healing and resilience.

The traumatic experiences that African Americans have faced throughout history, such as slavery and racial discrimination, can have a direct effect on mental health issues. Research has shown that trauma can interfere with the brain's capacity to respond to stress in an adaptive manner. This can manifest in various psychological difficulties, such as depression, anxiety, and post-traumatic stress disorder (PTSD), among others. Trauma further disrupts the ability of individuals to regulate emotions and engage in positive behavior that supports their overall well-being.

The physical effects of trauma are also important to consider when looking at its impact on mental health. Exposure to violence and other types of trauma can cause long-term physiological changes that affect the body's functioning. These changes may include chronic headaches, stomach aches, and other physical ailments. Additionally, individuals may experience difficulty with sleep, concentration, and memory.

The effects of trauma may also extend to the social realm. Trauma can make it difficult for individuals to maintain relationships, particularly if they feel disconnected or ashamed of their experiences. People who have experienced trauma may be more likely to engage in risky behavior, such as substance abuse, due to feelings of shame or guilt associated with their traumatic events.

Further, when looking at the impact of trauma on mental health, specifically among African American communities, access to mental health services is an important factor that should be taken into consideration. Research shows that there are disparities in access to mental health care for African Americans compared to other racial groups, which impedes recovery from trauma and other mental health challenges.

Finally, it is important to recognize that not all African Americans will experience the same effects of trauma on their mental health. This is due to differences in individual resilience, access to resources and supports, as well as the type and intensity of traumatic events experienced. It is therefore necessary to provide tailored interventions that are specifically designed for each individual's unique needs.

Recognizing the Signs of Trauma in Individuals and Families

When it comes to recognizing the signs of trauma in African American communities, it is important to be aware that not all people will experience or display their reactions to trauma in the same way. Therefore, it is essential for those providing services and support to individuals and families to be aware of the common signs of trauma.

One of the most telling signs that an individual has been exposed to a traumatic event is changes in behavior. These may include avoiding activities or situations which are associated with the traumatic event, engaging in self-destructive behavior, such as substance abuse, or displaying outbursts of anger. Other signs to look out for include difficulty with sleep, concentration, and memory; changes in eating habits; feelings of hopelessness or helplessness; and physical symptoms, such as headaches or stomachaches.

It is also important to recognize the signs of trauma in families. When a family member has been exposed to or experienced a traumatic event, there may be changes in family dynamics, such as increased conflict between family members, decreased communication, and disruption of roles within the family unit. Furthermore, parents may struggle with providing support to their children due to their own mental health issues associated with trauma exposure.

When recognizing the signs of trauma in individuals and families, it is also important to be aware of any cultural differences that may impact how they express their experiences. For example, African Americans may not feel comfortable talking about their traumatic experiences due to stigma around mental health issues or the fear of judgment from their peers.

This can make it more difficult for those providing services and support to recognize when an individual is struggling with the effects of trauma.

It is therefore important to create a safe space where individuals and families can openly discuss their experiences without judgment or shame. This will allow them to get the help they need while also giving service providers the opportunity to offer appropriate interventions and support.

Understanding How Trauma Can Be Passed On Intergenerationally

When looking at the impact of trauma on African American communities, it is important to understand that the effects can go beyond those who are directly exposed to traumatic events or experiences. That is because trauma can be passed down intergenerationally, meaning that its impact can extend even further than those who experience it directly.

Intergenerational trauma is defined as the transmission of emotional and psychological pain from one generation to the next, often due to traumatic experiences, such as slavery, genocide, war, or institutionalized racism. It can manifest in different ways, such as physical and mental health issues, economic instability, or even substance abuse. In African American communities, this trauma has been passed down for generations due to the history of discrimination and oppression they have faced.

This intergenerational transmission of trauma is especially prevalent when it comes to the effects of slavery on African Americans. Empirical studies have shown that the psychological effects of slavery—such as PTSD, depression, and anxiety—are still present in the African American community today. This is because these psychological issues are often passed down through families via stories and narratives about their lived experiences with oppression.

Additionally, research has found that traumatic events among African Americans can lead to an increased risk of developing chronic diseases, such as diabetes or heart disease. While most of these diseases are caused by lifestyle choices, they could also be linked to the psychological stress associated with intergenerational trauma.

Intergenerational trauma can also manifest in the form of learned behavior or coping mechanisms that have been passed down through generations. For example, African Americans may have learned coping mechanisms, such as avoidance or passivity, from their ancestors in order to survive. While these coping strategies might have been helpful for survival in the past, they can be detrimental in contemporary society and can lead to further mental health issues.

The effects of intergenerational trauma are not confined to just one generation but rather can extend across multiple generations. This means that understanding how it is transmitted and addressing its effects is especially important in African American communities. It is therefore essential for individuals to recognize how this trauma may affect them and take steps to address its effects on their lives.

Finally, it is important to recognize the importance of resilience when looking at intergenerational trauma. Despite the difficulties that this type of trauma can bring, African American communities have shown remarkable resilience in the face of adversity. This is partially due to their strong sense of community and cultural bonds, which have enabled them to find strength and support even in the most difficult times.

The Relationship Between Trauma and Substance Abuse

Trauma and substance abuse often go hand in hand in African American communities. Traumatic experiences can lead to substance abuse, and conversely, substance abuse can increase the likelihood of experiencing further trauma. Understanding the mutual connection between trauma and substance abuse is essential for fostering resilience in African American communities.

There are several possible explanations for why this relationship exists between trauma and substance abuse. For one thing, people who experience trauma may turn to drugs or alcohol in order to cope with their pain. This is commonly referred to as "self-medicating" and can lead to a substance abuse problem. Additionally, individuals who are predisposed toward substance abuse may be more likely to be exposed to traumatic experiences due to their lifestyle choices. Additionally, the American criminal justice system has disproportionately targeted African Americans for drug offenses, which can lead to further trauma.

Substance use itself can also have a direct impact on mental health outcomes for those in African American communities. Substance abuse often comes along with its own set of traumas, such as violence and poverty, which can exacerbate pre-existing mental health issues. People who misuse substances may also be at an increased risk of developing psychiatric disorders or experiencing suicidal thoughts. Furthermore, substance abuse can lead to a decrease in functioning and motivation which can cause further stressors.

The impact of trauma and substance abuse on African American families is particularly concerning. Substance abuse within a family often leads to increased levels of financial and emotional stress for the entire family unit. This can be especially damaging for young children who have been exposed to trauma or other difficult experiences. Substance abuse increases the likelihood of domestic violence, neglect, and exploitation, which can all contribute to mental health problems in childhood and adulthood.

In conclusion, trauma in African American communities is an issue that cannot be overlooked. It has the potential to impact individuals and families on both a physical and psychological level, as well as pass down intergenerationally through generations. Furthermore, substance abuse often accompanies trauma which can further complicate existing mental health issues.

Recognizing the signs of trauma and providing tailored interventions for each individual's unique needs is essential for addressing this issue in African American communities. For those struggling with the effects of trauma or coping with substance abuse, reaching out for help is key to recovery. With access to proper resources and support systems, African Americans can find healing and resilience in the face of adversity.

CHAPTER THREE
PREVALENCE OF DIFFERENT MENTAL HEALTH CONDITIONS

Mental health conditions can be a tricky topic for many to discuss, especially in African American communities. However, it is critical that we approach the subject of mental health with openness and understanding if we are to foster healthier outcomes. In this chapter, we will explore different mental health conditions commonly seen in African American communities so that we may better understand how they might affect individuals and how to best address them.

We will cover topics such as depression, anxiety disorders, bipolar disorder, schizophrenia, post-traumatic stress disorder (PTSD), and substance abuse to get a better sense of the prevalence of each condition in the African American community. We'll also take a look at possible diagnostic methods and treatment options available for those living with any of these mental health conditions. It is our sincere hope that this information will serve as a useful resource for those dealing with the stigma of mental health in their own lives or the lives of their loved ones.

Common Mental Health Conditions in African American Communities

Mental health conditions are a reality for many people in the African American community, with depression, anxiety, bipolar disorder, schizophrenia, and post-traumatic stress disorder (PTSD) being some of the most commonly experienced conditions. It is important to understand these conditions so that individuals can seek appropriate help and support if needed.

Depression

Depression is an emotional, psychological, and physical condition that can be experienced by anyone at any age. In the African American community, depression is often overlooked or underdiagnosed due to the stigma surrounding mental health. This can lead to more serious long-term issues if left untreated; therefore, it's important that individuals recognize the signs of depression and seek the needed help.

Depression can manifest in various ways, such as a persistent feeling of sadness or loss of interest; changes in eating or sleeping habits; feelings of worthlessness and guilt; fatigue and lack of energy; difficulty concentrating or making decisions, and suicidal thoughts. It's important to remember that everyone will experience depression differently; therefore, it's significant to pay attention to your own feelings and emotions.

In African American communities, there are a number of cultural factors that can contribute to depression. Historical trauma and systemic oppression stemming from slavery, racism, and discrimination are some of the primary causes of depression in African American communities. Additionally, poverty and the lack of access to adequate health care can also lead to an increased risk of developing depression.

It's also important to note that depression can be exacerbated by certain lifestyle factors, such as poor nutrition, lack of exercise, and substance abuse. Additionally, those who experience a traumatic event or major loss may be more likely to develop depression. It's therefore imperative to be aware of these risk factors and take requisite steps to address them if necessary.

For those struggling with depression in African American communities, there are a number of treatment options available for you. Cognitive-behavioral therapy, which focuses on addressing unhealthy thought patterns and behavior, is often an effective form of treatment for depression. Additionally, medications such as antidepressants can be prescribed to help manage the symptoms of depression. It's important to consult with a qualified mental health professional before beginning any form of treatment for depression.

In addition to seeking professional help, there are also other measures that individuals can take to help manage symptoms of depression. Exercising regularly and engaging in activities that bring joy or stress relief can be beneficial. Additionally, maintaining strong social connections is important, as having a strong support system can make dealing with depression much easier.

By understanding the signs, risk factors, and treatment options for depression in African American communities, individuals can better equip themselves to recognize when they or their loved ones may be struggling. It's important to remember that seeking help is not a sign of weakness but rather a strength, and taking the first step toward seeking help can be an essential part of the healing process.

Anxiety

Anxiety can be an overwhelming feeling that can impact individuals of all ages and backgrounds, including those living within the African American community. Anxiety is often accompanied by physical symptoms such as increased heart rate, muscle tension, sweating, or difficulty breathing. It's important to recognize the signs of anxiety and take steps to address them if necessary.

Anxiety can be caused by a number of factors, including genetics, environment, lifestyle choices, and traumatic events. Many African Americans may suffer from more than one type of anxiety disorder, such as generalized anxiety disorder, social anxiety disorder, or panic disorder. Symptoms of these disorders can range from mild to severe and may include recurring worries, feelings of restlessness or being on edge, difficulty sleeping or concentrating, feeling detached from reality at times, and thoughts of death or suicide. Without treatment, symptoms can become worse over time.

Fortunately, there are a number of effective treatment options for anxiety in African American communities. Talk therapy or psychotherapy, is the most common form of treatment for anxiety and can provide individuals with tools to manage their symptoms. Cognitive Behavioral Therapy (CBT) is a type of talk therapy that focuses on changing thought patterns and behavior that may be contributing to anxiety.

Other therapies used to treat anxiety include exposure therapy, which involves gradually exposing an individual to their fears or anxieties in a safe environment; biofeedback, where individuals learn to recognize and control their body's physical reactions to anxiety-causing stimuli; and medications such as antidepressants or benzodiazepines.

If you think you may be experiencing symptoms of an anxiety disorder, the first step is to speak with your primary care physician or a mental health professional. The doctor will conduct an evaluation and determine if there are any underlying medical conditions that need to be addressed before initiating treatment. It is important to remember that anxiety is treatable, and there are numerous resources available for those living with it in the African American community.

Additionally, when seeking help, it is essential to work with a mental health professional who understands the unique cultural and social issues faced by African Americans. This will ensure that treatment is tailored toward addressing individual needs and provide resources for continued support after therapy ends. Finding the right therapist can make all the difference in managing anxiety symptoms.

Finally, it's important to remember that anxiety does not have to be a lifelong battle. With proper care and support, individuals living with anxiety can lead healthy and fulfilling lives. It's time for us as a community to break down the stigma of mental health and start talking about how we can better support one another. Together we can create an environment where those living with anxiety feel safe, supported, and empowered.

Bipolar Disorder

Bipolar disorder is a mental health condition that affects many individuals within the African American community. It is important to understand this condition and its associated symptoms so that individuals can receive proper treatment and support.

Bipolar disorder is characterized by periods of extreme highs and lows in mood, energy, and activity levels. During a manic episode, individuals may experience feelings of euphoria, increased energy levels, distractibility, impulsive behavior, risk-taking behavior, decreased need for sleep, or irritability. They may also have an inflated sense of self-importance or grandiosity. During a depressive episode, individuals may experience low moods, difficulty concentrating or making decisions, fatigue or lack of energy to complete tasks, changes in appetite leading to weight loss/gain, thoughts of suicide, and feelings of worthlessness or guilt.

The onset of bipolar disorder typically occurs during late teens and early adulthood but can start earlier in life or even later. If left untreated, bipolar disorder is a chronic condition with recurring episodes of mania and depression that may become more severe over time.

In the African American community, bipolar disorder can be challenging to diagnose due to several factors. These include differences in cultural norms and language, a lack of access to mental health services, and stigma surrounding mental illness. Additionally, it may be difficult for individuals from different backgrounds to recognize their own symptoms or understand how they are feeling due to cultural differences.

The treatment for bipolar disorder varies depending on the severity of symptoms and individual needs. Medication such as mood stabilizers, antipsychotics, antidepressants, anti-anxiety medications, and other drugs may be recommended by a physician to help manage symptoms. Additionally, psychotherapy and lifestyle changes such as regular sleep schedules, healthy diet, and stress management may be recommended.

Finally, it's essential for members of the African American community to understand that mental health conditions like bipolar disorder are common and treatable. By increasing awareness within the community about bipolar disorder and other mental health issues through educational initiatives, we can help reduce stigma and increase access to care so that all individuals can receive the help they need. With proper diagnosis and treatment, those living with bipolar disorder can live stable and productive lives.

Schizophrenia

Schizophrenia is a mental health condition that affects individuals from all backgrounds, including the African American community. It can present itself differently for each person, making it especially challenging to recognize and diagnose.

The most common symptoms of schizophrenia are delusions, hallucinations, disorganized thinking and behavior, and "negative" symptoms such as a lack of emotion or energy. Those living with schizophrenia may experience vivid hallucinations in the form of voices, people, or objects that are not real but seem to be present.

Delusions refer to false beliefs held by an individual that cannot be shaken despite evidence that it is untrue. Disorganized thoughts might include having difficulty concentrating or focusing on a task. Negative symptoms can include social withdrawal and diminished emotional expression.

Despite these challenges, it is possible to live a successful life with schizophrenia. So what does effective treatment look like? There are several medications available to treat schizophrenia, such as antipsychotics and mood stabilizers. In addition, psychosocial interventions like cognitive-behavioral therapy (CBT) have been found helpful in treating symptoms of the condition.

These challenges make it more important than ever for those living with schizophrenia and their loved ones to seek out support networks that understand their situation and provide resources that can manage the condition successfully. This could include support groups specifically built for individuals living with schizophrenia or organizations dedicated solely to helping those in the African American community manage a mental health disorder such as schizophrenia.

It is also important to remember that seeking help is not a sign of weakness but rather strength. Taking the first steps toward getting help can be an essential part of the healing process and can be life-changing for individuals living with schizophrenia.

Post-Traumatic Stress Disorder (PTSD)

Post-traumatic stress disorder, or PTSD, is a mental health condition that affects individuals in the African American community following a trauma. While anyone is at risk of developing PTSD, it is important to understand the unique factors which may increase an individual's susceptibility to this disorder.

Those who experience systemic racism and discrimination are more likely to experience traumatic events, which could lead to PTSD. This includes experiences such as police brutality, racial profiling, and other forms of violence and oppression. Additionally, those living in poverty or experiencing homelessness are also at increased risk due to their lack of resources and support networks.

The symptoms of PTSD can include flashbacks or nightmares related to the trauma; avoidance of activities or situations that remind them of the trauma; difficulty sleeping or concentrating; and feelings of guilt, shame, or despair. In severe cases, it can lead to suicidal thoughts or behavior.

Fortunately, there are several effective treatments for PTSD available in the African American community. Trauma-focused cognitive behavioral therapy is one of the most common forms of treatment that can help individuals process their trauma and learn skills to cope with their symptoms. This type of therapy can be used in both individual and group settings and often involves revisiting the traumatic event in order to better understand it.

In addition to talk therapy, medications such as antidepressants or anti-anxiety drugs may be prescribed by a physician to manage symptoms related to PTSD. It is important to seek treatment from a qualified mental health professional who has experience working with individuals from the African American community.

Diagnosing Mental Health Conditions: Challenges and Solutions

The diagnosis of mental health conditions within the African American community can be challenging due to several factors, including the lack of access to mental health services, cultural differences, language barriers, and stigma associated with seeking help. These challenges can lead to delayed or missed diagnoses of conditions such as depression, anxiety disorders, bipolar disorder, schizophrenia, and post-traumatic stress disorder (PTSD).

The good news is that there are solutions and resources available to help African Americans get accurate diagnoses and access the care they need. One of the most important first steps is to build trust between individuals and their care providers by being open, honest, and showing respect for cultural differences.

Another crucial step is educating individuals about all available resources, including local community mental health centers and national organizations that provide information on diagnosis and treatment. Additionally, healthcare providers should be aware of potential language barriers among patients so they can adjust their communication style accordingly.

In some cases, individuals may also benefit from second opinions or referrals to specialists. It's important to remember that seeking help is a sign of strength, not weakness. When it comes to mental health, early diagnosis and treatment are key components for achieving and maintaining overall well-being.

Technology can also play an important role in the diagnosis process. Many mental health conditions share similar symptoms with physical illnesses, so technology such as mobile apps and wearable devices can help healthcare providers monitor patients' vital signs in real-time and more accurately diagnose conditions such as depression, anxiety disorders, bipolar disorder, schizophrenia, PTSD, or substance use disorder.

Finally, it is essential to remember that the African American community needs to come together and fight the stigma associated with mental illness. By doing so, we can create an environment in which individuals feel more comfortable seeking help and accessing the care they need. We must continue to break down barriers to treatment and support one another on our paths toward healing. There is no shame in seeking help for a mental health condition—it is a sign of strength. With proper support, treatment, and self-care, those living with mental health conditions can lead healthy and fulfilling lives.

Different Types of Therapies

When it comes to mental health, there are many different types of therapy available to individuals from the African American community. These can include cognitive-behavioral therapy (CBT), dialectical behavior therapy (DBT), psychodynamic therapy, acceptance and commitment therapy (ACT), and family/couples counseling. It is important to understand each type of therapy before deciding which one is best for you or your loved one.

Cognitive Behavioral Therapy (CBT) is a form of talk therapy that focuses on identifying and changing negative thought patterns or behavior that may be causing distress. CBT has been found to be effective in treating a variety of mental health conditions, such as anxiety, depression, and post-traumatic stress disorder (PTSD).

Dialectical Behavior Therapy (DBT) is an evidence-based form of CBT that was developed to treat individuals with borderline personality disorder. DBT focuses on teaching skills such as mindfulness, emotion regulation, distress tolerance, and interpersonal effectiveness.

Psychodynamic Therapy is a type of talk therapy that aims to help individuals gain insight into their unconscious thoughts and behavior. This type of therapy has been found to be helpful in treating depression, anxiety disorders, PTSD, substance use disorders, and other mental health conditions.

Acceptance and Commitment Therapy (ACT) is a form of psychotherapy that helps individuals accept their thoughts, feelings, and behavior in order to create meaningful change. It is often used to treat anxiety, depression, PTSD, addiction, and other mental health conditions.

Finally, family/couples counseling can be a helpful tool in managing relationships between spouses or family members. This type of therapy can help individuals better understand one another's perspectives and work on communication strategies to resolve conflicts.

The stigma surrounding mental health conditions persists in many African American communities, but it is our sincere hope that this chapter has provided valuable insight into how these conditions can affect individuals and what resources are available to those who may be dealing with them. With knowledge comes power. Let us begin to use it to combat this stigma and create an environment where all African Americans can feel comfortable seeking the help they need.

We cannot talk about mental health without acknowledging the importance of self-care. It is essential that we practice self-care techniques when dealing with sensitive topics such as these, including proper rest, nutrition, exercise, and relaxation. Mental health should be viewed in a holistic manner—looking at physical, emotional, social, and spiritual aspects for a complete picture.

CHAPTER FOUR
CULTURAL RESPONSES TO MENTAL HEALTH

Mental health isn't something that you would typically discuss at a family reunion. So how do African American communities respond to mental health issues? It's an often overlooked topic in our culture and is one of the biggest sources of stigma. In this chapter, we'll explore how cultural norms, religious beliefs, family dynamics, and other factors can contribute to the stigmatization of mental health in African American communities as well as what can be done to address these issues.

It's important to recognize that while there may be certain commonalities between African American communities when it comes to addressing mental health topics, each community will have its own unique perspective on the matter. The focus of this chapter is to explore how these conversations are taking place and how we can help shift the dialogue in a positive direction. Let's dive into the cultural responses to mental health!

How Cultural Norms Impact Mental Health Conversations

Cultural norms can have a profound impact on conversations surrounding mental health, and this is especially true within the African American community. Stigma, mistrust, and personal weakness are common barriers when it comes to seeking mental health care, but cultural norms such as resilience, self-reliance, and collectivism can both support and hinder these efforts.

Stigma is a major factor when it comes to mental health in the African American community. Stigma can stem from various sources, such as historical trauma, cultural norms, religious values, media stereotypes, and a lack of education. This stigma can cause feelings of shame and embarrassment that may prevent individuals from seeking out much-needed professional help or adhering to treatment recommendations.

Mistrust is another barrier to seeking mental health care among African Americans. Mistrust arises from personal experiences of racism, discrimination, bias, mistreatment, or exploitation by healthcare professionals or institutions. Non-Black healthcare providers also often lack cultural competence and sensitivity, which can further compound these issues. Furthermore, there is limited access to quality mental health care in many areas, which creates trust issues with those who do have access.

Personal weakness is another barrier to seeking mental health care in the African American community. Personal weakness is the perception that mental illness is a sign of personal failure, flaw, or defect. This can be shaped by cultural norms that emphasize strength, resilience, self-reliance, and independence, as well as religious beliefs that attribute mental illness to a lack of faith, sin, or spiritual warfare, among others. These attitudes can discourage individuals from admitting their mental health problems, asking for help, or accepting professional assistance.

On the other hand, cultural norms such as resilience, self-reliance, and collectivism can both support and hinder mental health efforts in the African American community.

Resilience can be an important tool for individuals in the African American community to cope with adversity and enhance their overall well-being. This resilience is often seen as a positive trait that enables people to persist despite difficult challenges and circumstances. While this can certainly foster strength, courage, and determination, it can also have some negative impacts if taken too far. Unreasonable expectations of oneself or others can lead to feelings of anxiety or depression when these expectations are not met. Moreover, resilience can sometimes be used as a way to mask emotional distress from others, which can prevent individuals from seeking help and support.

Self-reliance can increase self-confidence and autonomy, but it can also reduce social support and increase isolation. This can be especially true for the members of the African American community who may feel that it is their responsibility to shoulder all of their own burdens. Self-reliance can also lead to an over-emphasis on individualism and a reduction in support networks, which are vital sources of connection and comfort when facing mental health challenges.

Collectivism is a powerful cultural norm that promotes togetherness, unity, and shared purpose within many African American communities. While this sense of connectedness can foster strength and resilience, it can also lead to suppressed feelings or emotions if individuals fear being judged by others when they express themselves openly. Furthermore, collectivism can create a culture of silence surrounding mental illness that further perpetuates stigma and denial within the community.

When it comes to conversations about mental health in the African American community, understanding these cultural norms is essential. It's important to recognize how they both support and hinder efforts at seeking professional help. Doing so will help individuals feel more comfortable talking about their mental health issues and more willing to seek out available resources. Mental health professionals should also strive to be culturally competent and sensitive in order to build trust with their patients and provide quality care that meets their needs.

The Role of Religion in Mental Health

Religion and spirituality are deeply intertwined concepts that can shape the identity and well-being of many African Americans. While religion refers to the organized beliefs, practices, and institutions that connect people to a transcendent reality, such as God or a higher power, spirituality relates to the personal, subjective, and experiential aspects of one's relationship with the divine or sacred.

Religion is central to the identity and well-being of many African Americans who identify with historically Black Protestant denominations such as Baptist, Methodist, Pentecostal, or AME churches that affirm their dignity, value, and agency as people of faith. Some African Americans also belong to other Christian traditions, such as Catholicism or Jehovah's Witnesses or non-Christian faiths like Islam or Buddhism. Religion provides a source of resilience, hope, and empowerment for African Americans throughout their struggles against slavery, oppression, discrimination, and violence. It also offers a framework for understanding and coping with suffering, injustice, and death.

Spirituality is also central to the identity and well-being of many African Americans because it reflects their personal connection to God or a higher power. It can help enhance self-esteem, self-awareness, and self-transcendence by providing a source of healing and coping mechanisms for those who face stressors like racism, trauma, violence, or poverty. Prayer, meditation, music, art, or social action are all ways in which African Americans express their spirituality. For some, spiritual practices may provide more flexibility and autonomy than organized religion.

The role of religion and spirituality in the mental health of African Americans can go both ways. On one hand, religion can provide a sense of solidarity and support among those who share common faith, traditions, and values. Black churches can serve as spaces for worship, fellowship, education, advocacy, and social service in their communities. Prayer can help reduce anxiety, depression, and anger among African Americans who experience discrimination or injustice. Religion also provides an ethical framework to live according to faith principles which often inspire efforts toward social justice, peace, and reconciliation.

On the other hand, religious beliefs may interfere with professional mental health care by conflicting with it or reinforcing stigma or self-blame. Some African Americans may avoid seeking help because they perceive it as a sign of weak faith or distrust of God. They may also face judgment from their religious community for having a mental health condition or using mental health services. Similarly, some may believe that their mental health problems are caused by punishment from God or personal sin, or moral failure and prefer to rely on prayer or spiritual healing rather than medication or therapy.

Religion can also interfere with mental health care in more subtle ways. For instance, religious teachings on morality and sin can lead to feelings of guilt, shame, or self-blame which can exacerbate feelings of depression or anxiety. Some African Americans may view seeking help as an act of disobedience or failure to trust God and be sufficiently devoted to their faith. Religious beliefs may also create a sense of fatalism that leads to passivity in the face of adversity instead of taking action on one's own behalf.

In addition, religious teachings may discourage the use of medication or psychotherapy, which can be essential for treating mental health conditions. Some African Americans who rely on prayer as their primary form of healing may not realize that medication and therapy can have an additional positive effect in helping to manage mental health issues. Furthermore, even when African Americans do seek professional help, they may feel uncomfortable discussing sensitive topics such as sexual orientation or gender identity due to religious beliefs about these issues.

However, religion can also support mental health care when African Americans view it as a way of honoring God's will or taking care of the body as His temple. Religious beliefs can enhance the effectiveness of the treatment when they are integrated into the process alongside a culturally and religiously competent provider. It is important to note that religious beliefs and practices can have different meanings for different individuals; therefore, having cultural sensitivity is crucial when providing mental health care to African Americans.

Ultimately, it's important to remember that faith and mental health are not mutually exclusive—they can coexist and even enhance each other. By opening up the dialogue and moving forward with compassion and understanding, we can start to shift away from stigma and toward acceptance.

The Power of Family Dynamics

The power of family dynamics in promoting stigma associated with mental health in the African American community cannot be understated. Family dynamics shape individual identity, values, beliefs, roles, expectations, communication styles, coping strategies and intergenerational trauma, which all influence how an individual approaches mental health challenges.

Family roles are an important part of family dynamics as they dictate the responsibilities and expectations of each family member. In some cases, these roles can be flexible and adaptive to changing circumstances, but in other families, they can be rigid and restrictive. For African Americans, this can often lead to a sense of inability to meet those role-based expectations either because of external stressors such as racism or poverty or due to internalized shame or guilt associated with not measuring up to those expectations.

Family expectations are also a key factor in family dynamics. These can be supportive and encouraging, leading to greater self-worth and belonging, or they can be demanding and critical, creating feelings of pressure, guilt, or shame. This often encourages individuals to internalize any negative emotions or behavior associated with mental health issues rather than seeking help from outside sources.

The way family members communicate is another important factor to consider when it comes to stigma related to mental health in the African American community. Healthy communication styles involve open dialogue among family members that encourages understanding and trust, while hostile communication styles lead to misunderstanding, conflict, and resentment. This can further discourage African Americans from seeking outside help for fear of being misunderstood or judged by their family members.

Family coping strategies are also a key factor in the promotion of mental health stigma. Positive and adaptive coping strategies involve reaching out to social networks, using humor, or relying on spirituality, while negative and maladaptive coping strategies involve avoiding or denying problems, blaming or scapegoating others, or abusing substances. These negative coping mechanisms often lead to greater isolation on an individual level which can lead to more internalized shame and guilt around the issue of mental health.

Intergenerational trauma is another factor that has been identified as a major contributor to mental health stigma in the African American community. This trauma is passed down from one generation to the next and can affect mental health by causing emotional pain, anxiety, depression, anger, or post-traumatic stress disorder (PTSD). Conversely, intergenerational trauma can also inspire resilience, strength, courage, or activism in individuals.

Family dynamics may either facilitate or hinder help-seeking and treatment adherence for mental health issues. Healthy family dynamics can provide emotional support, practical assistance, information, and referrals, while negative dynamics create barriers to seeking outside help. Additionally, healthy family dynamics reduce the stigma associated with mental health while reinforcing it using closed communication styles or demanding expectations.

The power of family dynamics in African American communities extends beyond conversations surrounding mental health—intersecting forms of oppression such as racism, sexism, homophobia, and other systemic issues can also impact how individuals perceive their mental health struggles.

For example, black men are often seen as hyper-masculine and are expected to adhere to traditional gender roles which emphasize strength and independence—any sign of vulnerability or weakness is discouraged. This can lead to feelings of shame among those struggling with their mental health who feel like they don't fit into the traditional definition of what it means to be a man.

Moreover, class and economic disparities can have a profound impact on how African American families view mental health issues. For example, individuals from low-income backgrounds may be more likely to experience stigma due to a lack of access to resources and services that could help them with their mental health struggles.

Additionally, those from lower-income households may not feel comfortable discussing their mental health condition due to fear of judgment or ridicule from family, friends, and peers. This could lead to feelings of shame and isolation which further exacerbate their mental health struggles.

Furthermore, class and economic disparities can prevent individuals from receiving the care they need due to financial constraints or an inability to access treatment options in their area. Those who live in rural or underserved areas may not have access to quality mental health services which can further compound their suffering.

It's also important to recognize the role of poverty in exacerbating mental illness. Those living in poverty are more likely to experience chronic stressors such as food insecurity, housing insecurity, and job instability which can all contribute to poor mental health outcomes. In addition, racism and other forms of systemic oppression can create additional barriers for individuals from low-income backgrounds when it comes to seeking out professional help for their mental health concerns.

In conclusion, it is clear that the stigma of mental health in the African American community is complex and multifaceted. It is a deeply-rooted issue, with cultural norms playing an important role in determining how individuals think about and respond to mental health issues. Moving forward, we must continue to work together as a community to break down these stigmas and reduce the suffering caused by mental illness. With increased support, education, awareness, and access to quality care, all members of our community can have improved access to resources and live healthier and more fulfilling lives. Let's end the silence around mental health now!

CHAPTER FIVE
ACCESS TO MENTAL HEALTH CARE

Mental health care can be elusive for many, but even more so in the African American community. With limited access to services that could provide relief from stigma and pain, it is no wonder that discussing mental health has not been an easy conversation for members of this group.

In this chapter, we will take a closer look at the challenges that have long plagued African American communities in getting access to mental health care and how these can be addressed. We'll also explore the unique ways stigma manifests itself in those unable to access services due to their lack of resources or their inability to pay for treatment. By understanding these obstacles, we can move forward in creating a more inclusive society where mental health is no longer perceived as something to be hidden away and swept under the rug.

Access to mental health care is a critical factor in promoting overall wellness, yet it remains an elusive goal for many African American communities. To provide more comprehensive assessments and treatments, we'll need to tackle the barriers that limit access to these services.

These accessibility barriers can be physical—such as transportation difficulties or a lack of availability of services in the local area - or cultural, including negative perceptions and a lack of trust in the mental health system. There may also be financial constraints, as many people cannot afford to pay out-of-pocket for necessary treatments. All of these factors can lead to decreased access to resources and the continued cycle of stigma.

Let's delve deeper to examine the various obstacles that inhibit access to mental health care in African American communities.

Economic Challenges and a Lack of Coverage

The economic challenges faced by African American communities are a major barrier to receiving mental health care. Many lack the financial resources needed to pay for treatment out-of-pocket. African Americans are more likely to be employed in low-wage jobs with few benefits, and even those who do have health insurance may lack adequate coverage for mental health care. Even when insurance does cover some services, copays can be too high to make it feasible.

Furthermore, many individuals cannot take time off of work for needed therapy sessions due to a lack of paid sick or vacation days. This contributes to a cycle of poverty that exacerbates the need for access to mental health services while simultaneously making it difficult to seek out this care.

Moreover, many African Americans may not qualify for government-funded mental health coverage. This can be due to various factors, such as changes in eligibility requirements or denial of coverage based on pre-existing conditions. For those who do receive coverage, the wait times for available appointments and services are often too long, leading to further delays in care or exacerbation of existing symptoms.

In addition to basic economic challenges, there are often additional financial and administrative hurdles for African Americans seeking mental health care. These can include high deductibles, a lack of transportation reimbursement for travel to appointments, or difficulty understanding the complexities of insurance paperwork and billing. All of these issues combine to further reduce access to mental health care.

Not only are African Americans less likely to have insurance, but they're also more likely to underutilize their coverage. This can be due to a variety of reasons, including a lack of awareness about available services or fear of stigma associated with seeking treatment. Even when individuals do decide to pursue services, it can be difficult for them to find a provider who is knowledgeable about cultural issues and provides quality care in a way that is sensitive and respectful.

These financial and administrative barriers can also lead to disparities in the quality of care African Americans receive. Consequently, a lack of access to mental health care can result in more severe symptoms, decreased ability to cope with stressors, and poorer outcomes overall. As a result, African

Americans are more likely to receive low-quality care than their white counterparts—even when they have insurance coverage.

Systemic Discrimination in Health Care Settings

Systemic discrimination can also be a major obstacle for African Americans seeking mental health care. Studies have shown that Black people are less likely to receive the same quality of care as their white counterparts. This is due to implicit bias among providers, which can lead to diagnosis and treatment disparities.

Implicit biases manifest in various ways—from microaggressions such as unprofessional language or comments about race to a lack of cultural awareness or insight into how racism impacts an individual's lived experience. These biases influence providers' decisions about who is referred for mental health services, what types of treatments are recommended, and even how comfortable a patient feels disclosing personal information.

These disparities can be seen both in treatment outcomes and in access to care. African Americans are less likely than their white counterparts to receive evidence-based treatments such as cognitive behavioral therapy (CBT) and psychopharmacology. Instead, they're more likely to be prescribed medication without getting the necessary counseling or other support needed to ensure success with the medications.

Furthermore, African Americans are more likely to be seen in emergency rooms or psychiatric hospitals instead of getting the care they need in an outpatient setting. This can lead to misdiagnosis and other complications related to not receiving comprehensive mental health care. In addition, many providers lack the cultural competency necessary to build a trusting therapeutic relationship. As a result, African Americans may be less likely to feel comfortable discussing their mental health issues with providers, leading to underdiagnosis and poorer outcomes.

Systemic discrimination can also lead to disparities in who is referred for mental health care. Research has found that Black people are more likely than White people to be referred for involuntary hospitalization or outpatient services without being given the opportunity to make an informed decision about their treatment. This contributes to distrust of the mental health system and further reduces access to resources.

Finally, systemic discrimination leads to unequal representation in the field of healthcare overall—from a lack of diversity among providers, administrators, and policymakers responsible for making decisions about access to services. This lack of diversity can lead to a perpetuation of the same systemic inequalities that are preventing African Americans from getting the mental health care they need.

Distance From Services and Transportation Issues

Distance from services is also a major barrier to receiving mental health care for African American communities. Many individuals lack access to providers who are knowledgeable about their unique needs and cultural context, which can be particularly difficult if they live far away from urban areas with larger Black populations.

Even when services are available nearby, transportation issues can be an obstacle to receiving the care needed. A lack of access to reliable public transportation or inability to afford private transport makes it difficult for many African Americans to get to appointments in a timely manner—leading to missed appointments, delayed care, and further exacerbation of symptoms.

On top of this, the costs associated with transportation are a financial burden for many individuals. Gas prices, car maintenance, and parking costs can add up quickly, making it difficult to afford the necessary trips to visit providers or attend group therapy sessions. This is especially true in rural areas where distances are greater, and there may not be reliable public transportation available.

The issue of distance from access to services further complicates access to care for African Americans who need mental health treatment but do not live near major urban centers. Many rural communities lack specialized clinics that provide culturally competent care—meaning that individuals must travel long distances to get the help they need.

Distance from services can have an impact on children in particular. When a child must travel long distances to receive treatment, it can be difficult for parents to take time off of work in order to accompany them. This can lead to missed appointments and gaps in care, potentially causing further harm if symptoms are not adequately addressed.

All of these issues contribute to the continued stigma surrounding mental health in African American communities. Distance from services creates an additional barrier that prevents those who need help from getting it—making it easier for people to suffer in silence and perpetuating the cycle of shame and negative stereotypes associated with mental illness.

Language Barriers as an Obstacle

Language barriers can also be a major obstacle for African American communities seeking mental health care. Many individuals may not speak English fluently, making it difficult to communicate with providers or understand the complexities of paperwork related to insurance coverage. This lack of understanding can lead to delays in treatment, inadequate care, or even denial of services altogether due to failure to meet requirements.

In addition, providers must be aware of the nuances of language that are specific to African American culture when providing care. There may be certain terms used within the community that are not found in mainstream psychological literature but may provide important insight into the patient's lived experience. Without an understanding of these cultural nuances, providers risk creating a barrier to care for African Americans seeking mental health services.

Language barriers can also be a barrier to seeking mental health services due to inadequate translation and interpretation. This is particularly true for immigrants from African countries, who may find it difficult to understand the language of their new country or express themselves accurately in it. Many providers lack the resources necessary to provide competent translations and interpreters, leading to miscommunication between patient and provider that can impede care.

In addition, many African Americans speak dialects of English that are distinct from standard American English. These dialects may incorporate regional slang and other cultural expressions that can be difficult to understand for providers who don't have a comprehensive understanding of the nuances of language used within the community. Without an appreciation of these various linguistic influences and their implications for communication, providers risk creating further barriers to quality care.

The lack of access to resources in languages other than English can also affect the quality of mental health care received by African Americans. Many individuals need help navigating insurance paperwork or understanding diagnosis codes but may not have access to accurate translations or interpreters capable of providing clear information in their native tongue. This can lead to confusion about what services are provided and the cost of treatment, therefore, creating yet another obstacle to receiving quality care.

Finally, language barriers can lead to misdiagnosis or inadequate treatment of mental health issues in African American communities. Without a full understanding of an individual's cultural background and experiences, it is difficult for providers to accurately assess their needs or provide evidence-based treatments tailored to an individual's specific circumstances. As a result, individuals may not get the care that they need—potentially worsening symptoms and leading to poorer outcomes overall.

Limited Resources in Underserved Communities

The lack of resources in underserved communities is another major factor contributing to mental health crises, particularly among African Americans. Not only are there fewer mental healthcare providers available in these communities, but also those who exist may not always provide quality care due to limited access to resources.

One of the most pressing issues facing underserved populations is the availability of specialty mental health services, such as psychotherapy or medication management. These services can be hard to come by for individuals living in rural areas or those without insurance or other financial means to afford them. Even in some urban areas, there may not be enough providers to meet the needs of all patients.

The lack of specialized mental health services often means that individuals have to rely on general medical practitioners for their care—many of whom do not have adequate training or requisite knowledge of mental health issues. This can lead to misdiagnoses and inadequate treatment plans, as well as a greater stigma surrounding mental illness within these communities as people struggle to find help.

Another issue facing underserved populations is the lack of resources devoted to mental health. Financial constraints often limit how much money can go toward providing quality services, and organizations that serve these communities are often stretched thin trying to meet demands. This leaves many individuals without access to much-needed treatment or support—leading to further exacerbation of symptoms or even a worsening of their condition over time.

There is also a lack of preventive care in many underserved communities, which can be particularly detrimental for those suffering from mental illness. Without access to early intervention strategies such as counseling or therapy, individuals may not get the help they need until their symptoms become more severe—making it more difficult and costly to treat them effectively.

Finally, there is a lack of education and awareness about mental health in many underserved communities. Without adequate information or resources, individuals may not be aware of the signs and symptoms of mental illness or know how to access care if they do need it. This further contributes to the stigma surrounding mental health issues, as well as increasing people's risk of developing more serious conditions without getting proper treatment.

Unclear Diagnosis and Treatment Plans

The lack of specialized mental health services can lead to unclear diagnosis and treatment plans for African Americans suffering from mental illness, further contributing to the stigma around seeking help. Without access to evidence-based treatments such as cognitive behavioral therapy (CBT) or psychopharmacology, individuals may not receive the care they need—leading to ineffective outcomes and poorer quality of life overall.

Inadequate training can also lead to inaccurate assessments and misdiagnoses among providers without specialized knowledge in mental health issues. General practitioners often rely on less comprehensive diagnostic tools than those used by psychiatrists or psychologists; therefore, individuals may not receive the most effective treatment for their condition. This can lead to ineffective outcomes or worsening of symptoms if their disorder is not properly identified and treated.

The lack of resources dedicated to mental health in underserved communities also means that there are fewer providers available who are knowledgeable about cultural contexts such as race, ethnicity, religion, or other aspects of an individual's identity. This can make it difficult for individuals to receive culturally competent care, as providers may not be familiar with the unique needs of those from different backgrounds. As a result, patients may find themselves feeling misunderstood or unvalued by their providers, further increasing the stigma around seeking help and potentially leading to poorer outcomes.

In addition, there are often fewer treatment options available in underserved communities due to the lack of specialized services. Without access to evidence-based treatments such as psychotherapy or medication management, individuals may be stuck, relying on unproven interventions that do not provide lasting relief from their symptoms. This can lead to frustration and feelings of hopelessness among those seeking help, making it more difficult for them to get the care they need and leading to an overall deterioration in their mental health.

Finally, without adequate resources devoted to mental health care, individuals may not receive the long-term support they need for recovery. This can include follow-up appointments with providers or access to community support services that provide ongoing guidance and assistance in managing symptoms. Without this type of care, many individuals may find themselves struggling to cope with their disorder on their own, further contributing to the stigma around seeking help and perpetuating negative stereotypes associated with mental illness.

The Fear of Renewed Discrimination Due to Seeking Help

The fear of renewed discrimination is another major factor contributing to the stigma surrounding individuals with mental health conditions in African American communities. Many individuals are hesitant to seek help for their conditions, fearing that they may face further mistreatment or discrimination if they do so. This is particularly true for those with past experiences of prejudice based on their race or ethnicity, making it difficult for them to trust providers or feel comfortable discussing their issues openly.

Discrimination can manifest itself in many ways when it comes to accessing care—from denial of services due to an individual's race or ethnicity to condescending attitudes from providers who don't understand an individual's cultural context. In addition, many African Americans may hesitate to discuss their symptoms due to the fear that they will be judged or seen as weak for talking about their mental health issues. This can further discourage individuals from getting the help they need, leading to poorer outcomes overall.

The fear of discrimination is linked to wider socio-economic factors, such as systemic racism and a lack of access to quality resources in underserved communities. As previously mentioned, many African Americans living in poverty have difficulty affording mental health care or are unable to access culturally competent providers due to limited services available in their area. This creates an additional barrier to seeking help, as individuals worry that they may not be taken seriously or respected by those providing care.

Additionally, African Americans may be hesitant to seek help due to distrust of the healthcare system as a whole. Many individuals have had negative experiences in the past with providers who did not take their concerns seriously or failed to provide adequate treatment. This makes them feel that their needs will not be met in the future. This fear can further exacerbate the stigma surrounding mental health and make it more difficult for individuals to get the help they need.

Many African Americans may also fear that seeking help for their mental health issues could lead to further discrimination or prejudice from those in the community. This is particularly true for individuals who have experienced past discrimination based on their race or ethnicity—as they worry that opening up about their struggles may invite judgment or ridicule. This can lead to a reluctance to talk about their issues openly and make it more difficult for them to receive care.

Though the stigma surrounding mental health in African American communities is a real and pressing issue, there are tangible steps that can be taken to ensure that individuals receive quality care. By increasing education and awareness about mental health issues, providing access to culturally competent providers, and creating long-term support systems for those seeking help, we can start to reduce the stigma associated with seeking treatment, ensuring that all individuals receive the care they need and deserve. With these efforts, we can work toward erasing the stigmas associated with mental health in African American communities and creating an equitable system of care for all.

CHAPTER SIX

OVERCOMING THE MENTAL HEALTH STIGMA

It's no secret that the stigma of mental health in African American communities can be a huge barrier to receiving the care and support needed. However, it doesn't have to be this way; there are steps we can all take toward breaking down the wall of mental health stigma. In this chapter, we look at how individuals, families, and communities can work together to combat the stigma and create healthier mental health outcomes.

From challenging misconceptions to creating a more supportive environment, there are numerous ways we can start reducing mental health stigma in African American communities. Even small steps can add up to big results! So let's get started on breaking down these barriers so everyone can have access to the care they need and deserve.

Challenging Popular Misconceptions and Myths

It's no secret that mental health stigma has held a strong grip on African American communities for far too long. But it doesn't have to stay this way; part of the solution involves challenging the popular misconceptions and myths surrounding mental illness. Only then can we start to create more positive outcomes and reduce stigma in our communities.

One of the first myths we need to challenge is that mental illness can be prevented or cured with willpower alone. This simply isn't true; mental illnesses are serious medical conditions that require professional treatment. Ignoring the signs and symptoms won't make them go away.

Another common myth is that people with mental illness are dangerous or violent; this isn't backed by evidence, and it perpetuates stigma while ignoring the fact that most people with a diagnosable mental illness are not violent. It's also important to recognize that seeking help for a mental health issue doesn't mean you have "failed" as an adult. In fact, it takes maturity and strength to admit when you need support from professionals who can help.

Another common myth is that mental health issues only affect people of a certain race or ethnicity. This couldn't be further from the truth; anyone can experience a diagnosable mental illness, regardless of their background. It's important to note that minority populations are often at higher risk for experiencing mental health problems due to various factors such as racism, poverty, and limited access to quality healthcare. So it's critical that we challenge this myth in order to create better understanding and reduce stigma in our communities.

It's also essential that we challenge the popular belief that medication is always necessary for treating mental illnesses. While medication can be beneficial for some people, it isn't always the best course of action; in many cases, cognitive behavioral therapy or other forms of talk therapy can be just as effective (if not more). It's important to understand that everyone's experience and needs are different, and there isn't a one-size-fits-all approach.

We need to challenge the idea that people with mental illness are somehow "less than" or "inferior." This belief is based on outdated stereotypes and prejudices—and it only serves to further stigmatize those who are already struggling. Instead, we should recognize that everyone has value regardless of their mental health status and celebrate those who have the courage to seek help for their issues.

Again, it's essential that we challenge the myth that mental health issues are something to be ashamed of. This isn't true; learning more about mental health can actually help reduce stigma and create a more supportive environment for those who need it most. Seeking help is nothing to be ashamed of—it means you care enough about yourself and your well-being to get the professional support you need.

Creating a Supportive Environment for Mental Wellbeing

Creating a supportive environment for mental well-being is key to reducing stigma in African American communities. By recognizing the signs of mental health issues, providing support to those who need it, and creating an atmosphere that's free from judgment and shame, we can help foster better understanding and create healthier outcomes for everyone involved.

One way to create a more supportive environment is to start conversations about mental health in our families, neighborhoods, places of worship, schools—basically anywhere people gather. This helps normalize the conversation around mental health so that individuals feel comfortable discussing their own issues and struggles, as well as those of their friends and family.

It's also helpful to learn more about mental health issues so we can better understand and appreciate what people are going through. This means taking the time to research different disorders, familiarize yourself with symptoms, and educate yourself on how different treatments work. Although it's not always easy for those who don't have a personal connection to mental illness, having an understanding and appreciation of these issues is essential for creating a supportive environment in which individuals feel comfortable seeking help.

We should also be willing to offer support whenever possible. This could mean checking in on someone who hasn't been around or providing resources for treatment if they need it. Simple acts of kindness can make a world of difference to someone who is struggling. It's also important to remember that everyone responds differently to treatment, so be sure to offer non-judgmental support and understanding as they navigate their own journey.

We need to create an atmosphere in which people don't feel ashamed or embarrassed about seeking help for mental health issues. This means reframing the conversation around mental illness and emphasizing that seeking help is a sign of strength rather than weakness. We can do this by celebrating those who take the brave step of admitting they need help and offering our own stories and lived experiences when appropriate.

It's important to remember that change takes time and effort. We can start by speaking up for those who don't have a voice or challenging popular misconceptions and myths about mental illness. We must also be willing to challenge our own beliefs and biases in order to create a more supportive environment. Only then can we start taking small steps toward reducing stigma in our communities.

Educating our Communities about Mental Health

Educating our communities about mental health is an essential step toward reducing the stigma against mental health conditions in African American communities. The more we learn, the better equipped we are to understand what individuals are going through and provide them with the support they need—without judgment or shame.

We can start by speaking out against discriminatory comments or language that marginalizes people who have a mental illness. This simple act can have a powerful impact on creating a more supportive environment and showing people that they aren't alone.

We should also take the time to educate ourselves about mental health issues so we can better understand what individuals are going through. This means doing some research on different disorders, familiarizing yourself with symptoms, and learning how different treatments work. We should also be willing to ask questions and learn more if someone opens up about their experience—this shows them that you care and want to help in any way possible.

It's also essential that we recognize the signs of mental health issues in our families, friends, and communities; this could mean anything from noticing changes in behavior or mood to speaking up when someone is engaging in risky behavior. By being aware of what's going on, we can start to create a more supportive environment and encourage individuals to seek help if they need it.

We must also be willing to challenge the popular misconceptions around mental health issues and speak up when these outdated beliefs are perpetuated. Only then can we begin creating better understanding and reducing stigma in our communities.

Finally, we must reach out to organizations that provide resources for those struggling with mental illness; this could mean anything from providing information about available treatments or services to connecting people with support groups or other helpful programs. There are numerous organizations out there working hard to promote understanding and acceptance—so be sure to take advantage of them!

Seeking Professional Help and Treatment

For many, seeking professional help for mental health issues can be difficult—especially in African American communities where stigma is still pervasive. However, it doesn't have to be this way; with the right support, treatment is available, and it can make a world of difference in improving mental well-being.

The first step toward seeking professional help for mental health issues is recognizing when you need it. It's essential to be aware of the signs and symptoms of different mental health disorders, as this can help you determine whether it's time to seek professional help. Common signs and symptoms of mental illness include changes in mood or behavior, feelings of hopelessness or worthlessness, difficulty concentrating, withdrawal from activities that used to bring joy, and thoughts of self-harm or suicide. If any of these apply to you (or someone you know), it's important to recognize them as early warning signs indicating that professional help might be needed.

It's also helpful to familiarize yourself with the various types of treatment options available—as this can make the process less overwhelming and intimidating. Talk therapy (also known as psychotherapy or counseling) is often beneficial for those struggling with mental health issues; this involves working with a trained professional who can provide support and guidance in negotiating through difficult emotions and life challenges. This type of treatment often focuses on developing coping skills, problem-solving strategies, and improving communication skills in order to better manage symptoms.

Medication is another option for those seeking treatment for their mental health issues; medications are typically prescribed by psychiatrists after assessing an individual's needs. These medications are designed to target specific brain chemicals that have been shown to impact emotions, thoughts, behavior, and physical functioning, and they can be useful tools for managing symptoms associated with certain conditions. However, medication should never be used without first consulting a qualified doctor. Only a medical professional can determine which medication(s) might best address your individual needs.

Aside from talk therapy and medication, there are various lifestyle changes that may be beneficial in treating mental illness, such as getting adequate sleep, eating healthy foods, exercising regularly (which can release endorphins that boost mood), engaging in creative activities like art or music (which can help reduce stress), spending time outdoors (which has been linked with improved wellbeing), building supportive relationships with family and friends, reducing alcohol consumption/drug use (which can worsen symptoms), and utilizing relaxation techniques like deep breathing or mindfulness meditation exercises (which have been proven beneficial for managing stress).

The next step is finding a professional who can provide quality care. This means researching different providers in your area and being sure to read up on their experience and qualifications. Be sure to ask enough questions during the initial consultation so you know exactly what type of help they offer—and don't be afraid to look elsewhere if you don't feel comfortable with the provider or their approach.

It's also beneficial to seek support from family and friends throughout the process; having someone there who can listen without judgment or pressure can make all the difference when facing difficult emotions or tough decisions. It can also be helpful to join a support group—these are typically safe spaces filled with others who understand what you're going through and can offer valuable advice and insight.

Remember that seeking help isn't something to be ashamed of; in fact, it's a sign of strength rather than weakness. We should take the time to celebrate those who have the courage to admit when they need assistance—this will help create a more supportive environment for everyone involved.

By taking these steps, we can start to create better outcomes for those seeking professional help and treatment. This means understanding the importance of seeking help, finding a provider who's right for you, reaching out for support from family and friends, and celebrating those who have taken the brave step of admitting they need it. With time and effort, we can make great strides toward reducing stigma in our communities.

Increase Funds and Resources for Mental Health Services

Increasing funds and resources for mental health services is essential to reducing the stigma associated with mental health conditions in African American communities. With adequate funding, we can provide individuals with better access to quality care and create healthier outcomes for everyone involved.

One way to increase funds is by creating initiatives that raise awareness about the importance of mental health services; this could mean anything from launching campaigns designed to educate people about signs and symptoms of mental illness or hosting fundraisers to benefit local community centers providing treatment options. We should also encourage our friends, family members, and neighbors to donate their time or money toward these causes; this shows people that mental health is an issue we collectively take seriously and gives us the opportunity to create a more supportive environment.

We can also reach out to organizations dedicated to helping those with mental health issues, such as NAMI (National Alliance on Mental Illness) or local mental health advocacy groups. These organizations are often actively working to raise funds for different initiatives and programs designed to help those struggling with mental illness—and by dedicating our time or donating our money, we can show our commitment to creating healthier outcomes in our communities.

Another viable option is lobbying legislators at the local, state, and federal levels; changes in policy can have a powerful impact on how resources are allocated for mental health services. This could mean advocating for increased funding for different programs or improved access to care. It's also important to make sure our elected officials are aware of the importance of mental health issues and the need for adequate resources—this will ensure that these issues aren't overlooked or forgotten.

We should also be willing to volunteer at organizations dedicated to providing quality care; this can range from offering support in group therapy sessions or providing technical assistance with websites/social media accounts. Any way we can provide assistance is valuable and helps create a healthier environment for everyone involved.

Finally, we should be willing to speak up when mental health services are underfunded or inaccessible; this could mean anything from being an active participant in local campaigns advocating for better access to care or writing letters to our elected officials. Small actions can have a powerful impact—so let your voice be heard!

Increasing funds and resources for mental health services isn't easy—but it's essential if we want to reduce stigma in our communities. By taking the time to commit our energy and resources to create healthier outcomes, we can make great strides toward reducing discrimination and improving the way society views mental illness. Let's work together and create a brighter future for everyone involved!

Working with Community Leaders to Advocate Mental Health

Working with community leaders to advocate mental health is an essential step toward reducing stigma in African American communities. By creating relationships between community organizations and individuals, we can start to create a better understanding and provide resources that benefit everyone involved.

One way to work with community leaders is by presenting information about mental illness at local schools or universities; this could mean anything from providing lectures on the signs and symptoms of different disorders or offering workshops discussing treatment options and available resources. This will help raise awareness about the importance of mental health services, which can go a long way toward reducing stigma in our communities.

We can also team up with businesses and organizations to host events or campaigns that promote mental health awareness; this could mean anything from hosting fundraisers to benefit local treatment centers or providing information about available services at local community centers. By creating these types of initiatives, we can start to normalize conversations around mental illness and create a more supportive environment for everyone involved.

It's also beneficial to reach out to churches and other religious institutions in the area; many of these organizations are actively working to support those struggling with mental illness and provide resources for those seeking help. By connecting with them, we can make sure individuals are aware of the different services available and ensure they have access to quality care if needed.

Working with local politicians is another great way to advocate mental health; this could mean anything from connecting them with organizations providing resources or speaking out in support of better access to care. By doing this, we can start to create an environment that values mental health and emphasizes the importance of seeking quality treatment.

Finally, it's essential to create relationships with healthcare providers in the area; by forming partnerships between individual physicians and community centers, we can ensure individuals have access to quality care when they need it most.

This includes making sure providers are aware of the different treatment options available (such as medication or talk therapy) and educating them on how best to address certain issues/concerns their patients may be dealing with.

Creating Safeguards Against Discrimination and Racism

Creating safeguards against discrimination and racism is essential for reducing stigma in African American communities, as this can lead to improved access to mental health services and create better outcomes for everyone involved.

One way to do this is by encouraging open conversations about race and mental health and by having frank discussions about the challenges faced by individuals of color, we can start to create an environment that is more understanding of their needs. This means listening without judgment or criticism when someone shares their story—and being willing to acknowledge our own biases so we can be more aware of how they might have an impact on our behavior.

It's also helpful to familiarize ourselves with the different types of discrimination and racism individuals may experience; this could mean anything from reading up on the history of systemic racism or educating yourself about microaggressions. By understanding what these forms of oppression look like, we can start to create a more equitable environment for everyone involved.

Creating safeguards also means advocating for better services and access to care; this could mean anything from lobbying legislators at the local, state, and federal levels for increased funding or speaking out in favor of improved access to quality mental health treatment options. We should also be willing to volunteer our time at organizations providing resources, as this will help ensure those who need it have access to the care they need.

It's also important to reach out to local healthcare providers and make sure they are aware of the different needs of individuals of color; this could mean anything from ensuring physicians are educated on how best to provide culturally competent care or connecting them with community resources that can help address those issues. By doing this, we can start to create an environment that is more supportive and accommodating for everyone involved.

Finally, it's essential to support organizations that are actively working to reduce stigma in African American communities; this could mean anything from donating money or time to initiatives designed to provide better resources or speaking out when we see discrimination and racism occurring. By taking these steps, we can create a more equitable environment for everyone involved.

Overall, there are many steps we can take to reduce stigma in African American communities when it comes to mental health. From increasing funds and resources for mental health services to creating safeguards against discrimination and racism, we can create a healthier environment for everyone involved. It won't be easy—but with dedication and commitment, we can make great strides toward creating a society that values mental health and provides quality care for those who need it. Let's roll up our sleeves and get to work!

CHAPTER SEVEN

CULTURAL COMPETENCY OF MENTAL HEALTH PROVIDERS

Culturally competent mental health providers are critical in providing quality care to the African American community. Unfortunately, many mental health professionals lack the requisite knowledge and skills related to understanding, respecting, and responding effectively to cultural differences. In this chapter, we will discuss how mental health providers can better serve the African American community by becoming more culturally competent.

In order to be effective in treating African Americans with mental health issues, it is important that clinicians understand and respect the cultural backgrounds of African Americans. This includes being aware of cultural prejudices, biases, values, beliefs, and practices that might play a role in a patient's overall recovery process. Mental health professionals must also be prepared to address any disparities or stigmas associated with certain cultural groups when providing care. Finally, the cultural competency of mental health providers involves understanding the unique challenges faced by African Americans living in the United States and how those factors can affect their mental health.

The Importance of Understanding the Unique Cultural Experiences

It is essential for mental health providers to be culturally competent in order to provide effective care. Cultural competence is defined as the ability of a provider to effectively work with, understand, and appreciate individuals of diverse backgrounds. This requires an understanding of the core values, beliefs, language, religious practices, and historical experiences that may shape an individual's view of mental health care. For African Americans, cultural competency includes being aware of how systemic racism and oppression have impacted access to quality care over the years.

Culturally competent mental health providers are critical in providing quality care to the African American community. By understanding the unique cultural experiences and challenges of African Americans, mental health professionals can better serve this population. To become culturally competent, it is important that clinicians understand and respect the cultural backgrounds of African Americans.

One of the most significant differences between white Americans and African Americans is history. White Americans have had centuries to build upon their economic and social power, while African Americans continue to grapple with the effects of slavery and systemic racism. It is important for mental health clinicians to be aware of this distinct difference in order to better empathize with patients' perspectives and provide more effective treatment plans. Additionally, recognizing the direct influence historical events have on current-day circumstances can help clinicians better understand why some African Americans may be more likely to experience mental health issues.

It is also important to recognize the disparities in physical and mental health care that African American communities face. Systemic racism has resulted in unequal access to quality healthcare, leading to higher rates of premature death, poor disease management, and inadequate preventive services among African Americans. Mental health providers must be aware of these disparities when providing care so they do not further perpetuate existing inequalities.

Cultural competency requires a knowledge of the unique psychological stressors experienced by African Americans as well. The experiences of discrimination, poverty, violence, oppression, and exclusion result in an increased risk for mental health problems such as depression or anxiety disorders. By understanding the unique psychological stressors faced by African Americans, mental health providers can develop better strategies to meet their needs.

Mental health clinicians must also be aware of the stigma associated with mental illness in the African American community. Unfortunately, many African Americans believe that seeking help for a mental health issue is an admission of weakness or failure and thus feel ashamed to seek treatment. Therefore, mental health professionals must strive to create safe spaces where these individuals can feel comfortable expressing themselves and receiving help without judgment.

Finally, it is important for mental health providers to understand the unique cultural values and beliefs that many African Americans adhere to. These include respect for tradition, community-oriented approaches to problem-solving, and the belief that suffering can be spiritually meaningful. Being familiar with these values allows clinicians to provide more sensitive care tailored to their patient's needs.

Addressing Disparities or Stigmas Associated with Certain Cultures

Mental health providers must be prepared to address any disparities or stigmas associated with cultural groups when providing care. The first step is to become familiar with the particular challenges faced by members of these cultural groups, such as those experienced by African Americans discussed above. By understanding these experiences, mental health professionals will be better equipped to recognize the unique needs of their patients.

The second step is for clinicians to treat all patients equally and with dignity and respect regardless of their race, ethnicity, gender identity, or religion. This means respecting and honoring cultural differences without judgment. Mental health professionals should strive to provide services that are free from bias and discrimination, as well as create an environment where diverse perspectives can be heard and respected.

The third step is to develop a culturally competent treatment plan for each individual patient. This includes taking into account values, beliefs, practices, language barriers, and lifestyle in order to ensure the best possible care is provided. It also involves tailoring the treatment approach to meet the specific needs of the patient in order to maximize its effectiveness.

Mental health providers should proactively address any stigmas associated with certain cultures. This includes educating the public about the importance of seeking help for mental health issues and dispelling any negative stereotypes that are associated with members of certain cultural groups. Mental health professionals can also work directly with members of these communities to provide education and resources that will help reduce the stigma and encourage treatment-seeking behavior.

Finally, mental health providers must be committed to advocating for members of marginalized communities and addressing issues related to access and resources. This includes working with local organizations or institutions to provide culturally competent care and services, as well as developing collaborations with community leaders in order to increase awareness about mental health issues. Mental health professionals should also strive to ensure that all patients have equal access to quality mental healthcare regardless of their race, ethnicity, gender identity, or religion.

Providing Respectful Care to Diverse Populations

Mental health providers should strive to build trust with their patients by creating a safe space where people feel heard and respected. Providers should take the time to get to know their patients beyond what is noted on intake forms or in a diagnosis. This includes understanding patients' values, cultural and religious beliefs, and experiences with the health care system. Providers should also be aware of the unique challenges that African Americans face when accessing mental health services, such as financial barriers or stigma in seeking help in their communities.

In order to provide respectful care to diverse populations, providers must understand how power dynamics can impact a patient's experience. It is important for providers to ask questions in an open-ended way rather than assuming that all African American patients have similar experiences with mental illness. Providers should also avoid making unfounded assumptions about someone's culture based on outward appearances, such as language or clothing choices. In addition, providers should take time to learn about the different cultures and religions of those they work with, as well as any historical experiences that may have shaped an individual's view of mental health care.

In addition, providers should strive to create a culturally sensitive environment by using language and terminology that is respectful and appropriate. This includes avoiding denigrating words such as "crazy" or "insane" when referring to someone's mental illness. Providers should also be aware of how patient privacy is managed in order to preserve trust between the provider and the patient.

Furthermore, providers should understand the importance of providing holistic care that addresses both the physical and mental health needs of individuals. This includes taking into account all aspects of an individual's life, such as family, work, education, finances, spiritual beliefs, etc., when assessing their overall well-being. Providers should strive to provide comprehensive care that is tailored to each patient's specific needs and preferences.

In order to create a positive environment for African Americans accessing mental health services, it is important that providers take a collaborative approach that includes getting feedback from patients about their experiences with care. This can include surveys or focus groups as well as an open dialogue between providers and patients. Providers should also take the time to learn policies or regulations that may enhance their ability to provide quality care.

Incorporating Cultural Practices into Treatment Plans

When it comes to mental health care, it is imperative that providers strive to tailor treatment plans that will be most effective for their patients, which includes incorporating cultural practices when appropriate. Culturally sensitive care takes into account the values, beliefs, language, religious practices, and historical experiences of an individual's culture. This allows the provider to better address any unique challenges that a patient may face due to their cultural background as well as develop more effective strategies for treating mental health illnesses.

Incorporating cultural practices into treatment plans can involve a variety of approaches depending on the specific needs of the patient. This includes using appropriate and respectful language as well as accommodating any religious beliefs or dietary restrictions. Providers should also be aware of any special vacations or events that might impact a patient's treatment plan, such as a religious ritual or fast.

Again, providers should understand how historical events and systemic racism have impacted access to quality healthcare for African American communities over the years. The history of slavery, Jim Crow laws, and segregation has resulted in a long-standing racial inequality that continues to exist today. This has had a direct impact on access to healthcare for African American communities, leading to disparities in treatment and care.

For example, African Americans are more likely than white Americans to lack health insurance coverage as well as experience poorer quality care when they do receive it. This can mean longer wait times for appointments or less access to specialized care such as mental health services. Additionally, due to higher levels of poverty within the African American community, individuals may be unable to afford the necessary medications or treatments needed to manage chronic conditions or mental health illnesses.

Systemic racism has also led to disparities in educational opportunities which can further limit access to quality healthcare. Racial segregation historically limited opportunities for African American students, which can lead to lower academic achievement and fewer job prospects. Consequently, this affects the ability of individuals within these communities to gain meaningful employment with good health benefits or have the financial resources needed for medical expenses such as mental health services.

Incorporating cultural practices into treatment plans can involve utilizing traditional healing methods such as talking circles or spiritual ceremonies when appropriate. For example, some individuals may find solace in participating in a religious ritual or seeking the advice of an elder within their community.

Other approaches may include incorporating music therapy, art therapy, or mindfulness practices into treatment plans.

It is also important for providers to be aware of any cultural taboos when treating individuals from certain cultural backgrounds. For example, in some cultures, it may be inappropriate to discuss topics such as mental health or sexuality with someone outside of the family. It is essential for healthcare providers to take these sensitivities into account and respect cultural boundaries while still providing necessary care.

Finally, providers should strive to create treatment plans that emphasize the strengths of the individual rather than focusing solely on their illness. This includes recognizing and honoring the resilience of individuals who have survived despite facing significant challenges. Mental health providers can help empower their patients by celebrating these unique strengths and using them as a foundation for recovery.

Developing a Self-Awareness of Own Biases and Strengths

Providing quality care to patients from diverse backgrounds requires mental health providers to understand their own biases and strengths as well as the unique challenges faced by certain cultural groups. This includes recognizing any implicit or explicit biases they may have regarding race, ethnicity, gender identity, religion, or other social identities when interacting with patients. Additionally, it is essential for providers to understand how power dynamics can impact the patient's lived experience.

Developing self-awareness of own biases and strengths starts by recognizing any unconscious or conscious prejudices one may have toward certain cultural groups. This includes being honest and open about any preconceived notions or assumptions that one may have, as well as taking the time to educate oneself on different cultures and religions. Mental health professionals should strive to be aware of their own experiences, backgrounds, and privileges that may shape how they interact with members of diverse populations.

It is important for mental health providers to practice self-reflection in order to assess any potential areas of bias within their practice. This can include examining how often they refer patients from certain racial or ethnic backgrounds to specialists, how long wait times are for appointments, or the types of questions they ask when gathering patients' data. Taking an honest and unbiased look at these areas can help providers become more aware of their own biases and strengths as mental health providers.

Providers should also be mindful of how power dynamics can play a role in interactions with patients from marginalized communities. This includes understanding how language choices and body language can either foster or hinder a trusting relationship between the provider and the patient. For example, using overly technical terms with someone who has limited English proficiency can be detrimental to building trust, while using informal language with someone from a higher socio-economic status could demonstrate disrespect. Mental health professionals should strive to use respectful and appropriate language in every interaction in order to foster positive relationships with their patients.

Providers must also recognize that they may need to adjust their approach depending on the individual needs of each patient. This includes being aware of language barriers and utilizing interpreters when necessary, accommodating dietary restrictions, incorporating traditional healing methods into treatment plans, and adhering to any religious beliefs or practices. Providers should strive to create an environment where patients feel heard and respected regardless of their cultural background.

Additionally, providers should be aware of any systemic issues or policies that may affect access to quality mental health care for certain populations. This includes understanding how poverty, education levels, and employment opportunities can limit access to healthcare as well as advocating for policy changes that will provide equal access to quality care for all individuals.

It is important for mental health providers to remember that each individual's experience will be shaped by their unique values, beliefs, and practices within their culture—and these must be respected when providing care. By taking the time to develop an understanding of one's own biases and strengths, as well as those faced by members of diverse populations, mental health professionals will be able to provide more culturally sensitive care tailored specifically for each patient's needs.

By developing cultural competency, mental health providers can better serve the African American community and provide more effective care to individuals with mental health issues. Taking the time to understand the unique cultural experiences and challenges faced by African Americans is essential for providing quality services that meet their needs. It also opens up new pathways for building trust with patients from diverse backgrounds and increases access to inclusive forms of treatment. Ultimately, understanding and respecting different cultures can help create an environment of healing for all those in need of mental health care.

CHAPTER EIGHT
STRATEGIES FOR IMPROVING ACCESS TO MENTAL HEALTH CARE

Tackling the stigma of mental health in the African American community is a huge challenge that requires an effective strategy. One way to improve access to care and reduce this stigma is by introducing strategies that provide better services, more resources, and increased outreach to those who need it most.

This chapter looks at ways we can make strides toward improving access to mental health care in African American communities. We'll explore how funding for treatment can be improved, how transportation barriers can be broken down, and how language barriers can be reduced or eliminated. Additionally, we'll discuss having services tailored specifically for individuals living with mental health conditions, as well as other thoughtful approaches that could help eradicate the stigma associated with seeking mental health support. With these strategies in place, we can start to make a difference in African American communities and ensure those who need it receive the necessary care. Let's get started!

Increasing Funding for Mental Health Treatment

We cannot talk about improving access to mental health care without discussing increasing funding for the necessary treatments. All too often, African American communities are overlooked when it comes to funding for mental health services, leaving many without the resources they need to get quality care.

Fortunately, there are proactive steps that can be taken to ensure African Americans have access to the treatment they need. First, it is essential to advocate more funding on a local level. This means reaching out to city or county representatives in order to make them aware of the mental health needs in the community and how increased funding could help meet those needs. It is also essential to seek out grants from both public and private sources, as these can be valuable resources for mental health services in African American communities.

It's important to make sure that funding for mental health care is used wisely. To do this, it's beneficial to create an advisory committee that consists of individuals or organizations who are familiar with the needs of the local community. This committee can help ensure that funds are allocated appropriately and directed toward the areas where they are most needed. Additionally, it's important to track how funds are being used to ensure they are tailored toward the programs that will have the most impact.

However, increased funding for mental health care isn't just about money. It's also essential to make sure those who need treatment can access it without facing financial hardship. To do this, it is important to ensure that insurance companies are covering necessary treatments, such as therapy or medication. Additionally, providing low-cost or free services for those in need is an invaluable way of making sure African Americans don't encounter financial barriers when seeking treatment.

Finally, it's important to ensure that funds are used toward creating better mental health environments. This can include hiring more culturally competent staff, providing training on mental health issues specific to African Americans, and making sure practitioners understand the nuances of dealing with trauma within these communities. Additionally, it is essential to make sure resources are reaching African American communities in rural areas or other underserved locations.

By increasing funding for mental health treatment and ensuring that those who need help have access to care without financial hardship, we can start to make a difference in the lives of those living with mental health conditions in African American communities. With this increased Investment comes increased hope that everyone will be able to receive the quality care they deserve.

Improving Transportation Options

One major challenge for African Americans seeking mental health services is transportation. Oftentimes, individuals are unable to find reliable or accessible means of travel to get them to their appointments. This problem can be especially difficult for those who live in rural areas without access to public transportation or those with limited economic resources that cannot afford a car or taxi ride.

Fortunately, there are some strategies that can be implemented to improve transportation options for those seeking mental health services. One way is to provide them with access to transport vouchers or other forms of financial assistance that cover the cost of travel. This could include providing free rides through programs such as Lyft or Uber or partnering with local taxi companies to offer discounted fares for individuals in need.

Another option is to partner with public transport service providers to create a special program specifically designed for those who need help accessing mental health services. This could involve offering discounted rates or free passes on buses or trains that go directly to mental health facilities. Additionally, providing shuttle services from certain areas to specific destinations can also make it easier for African Americans living with mental illness to get to where they need to go.

In addition to providing transportation options, it's also important to ensure that they are safe and comfortable for those using them. This means avoiding overcrowded buses or trains and making sure the vehicles are regularly maintained and serviced. Additionally, having a clear wayfinding system in place can help reduce confusion when it comes to navigating unfamiliar routes.

Increasing awareness of available transportation options is essential. Educating organizations, service providers, and the public on available resources can make a huge difference when it comes to helping African Americans access mental health services. This could include creating informational flyers or other materials that explain how to use public transportation, partnering with local media outlets to spread the word, and even providing onsite training for those in need.

Finally, having a dedicated contact person or team who can provide guidance and support to those accessing these services can also make a difference. This could involve having someone available to answer questions about how to use public transportation or offering assistance with filing out paperwork for vouchers or discounts.

Improving access to mental health care requires thoughtful strategies that consider all aspects of the issue, including transportation options. By increasing awareness of available resources, making sure they are safe and comfortable, and providing additional forms of assistance when needed, we can help ensure African Americans have better access to the treatment they need without worrying about how they'll get there.

Reducing Language Barriers

Language barriers have long been a major obstacle to providing quality mental health care for African American communities. In many cases, Black Americans present symptoms of depression, anxiety, or other mental health issues that are not fully understood by healthcare providers who do not speak the same language. This is especially true when it comes to immigrant and refugee populations, as preconceived biases can lead to misdiagnoses or the neglect of treatments that would address underlying problems.

To overcome this challenge, more organizations need to make an effort to ensure their staff reflect the diversity of their patients and provide interpreters for non-English speaking clients. There has been a growing trend toward hiring bilingual therapists in recent years, which can help bridge communication gaps between provider and patient. Additionally, providers can invest in language-training tools such as an audio library of frequently used therapy terms and phrases or visual aids like charts and diagrams that illustrate key concepts.

It is also important to make sure that healthcare facilities are equipped with materials that explain mental health services in the patient's native language. This includes brochures, pamphlets, and any other printed material needed to clearly communicate treatment plans and expectations for each individual client. Furthermore, it is essential to ensure that staff members can speak the same languages fluently so they can respond quickly to questions or concerns from patients who do not understand English.

There are a number of online tools that can help make mental health care more accessible for those with limited English proficiency. For example, many providers now offer virtual counseling sessions through video conferencing software such as Skype or FaceTime. This allows patients to get the support they need without having to leave their homes or worry about language barriers. Additionally, several organizations have launched mobile apps that provide resources in multiple languages and allow users to connect with therapists who speak their native language.

Another strategy is to partner with local organizations that provide free translation services or cultural competency training for healthcare providers. For instance, some cities have established programs that pair immigrant mental health professionals and bilingual counselors with African American patients who do not speak English. This helps to promote better understanding between the provider and the patient while also ensuring that all conversations are conducted in a language both parties can understand.

Finally, it is important to create an inclusive environment within healthcare settings so that individuals from different backgrounds feel comfortable discussing their issues without feeling judged or misunderstood due to language barriers. This means providing interpreters when needed, making sure materials are available in multiple languages, and offering culturally appropriate services such as traditional healing modalities or group therapy sessions tailored to the patient's specific cultural needs.

Reducing language barriers is a critical part of making mental health care more accessible to African American communities. By investing in translation tools, hiring bilingual staff members, partnering with local organizations, and creating a welcoming environment, providers can help ensure that all individuals have access to quality care regardless of their background or native language. With these steps in place, more people will be able to get the support they need to lead healthier lives.

Utilizing Technology to Access Mental Healthcare

Technology has revolutionized the way people access mental health care, making it easier to connect with providers and receive treatment from the comfort of their own homes. This is especially beneficial for African American communities who may not have access to mental health services due to distance or financial constraints. By utilizing technology, more individuals can get the help they need without worrying about facing discrimination or the stigma associated with seeking help from traditional sources.

One popular form of technology-based mental health care is telemedicine, which involves providing counseling sessions over video conferencing platforms such as Skype or FaceTime. This allows patients to meet with their providers from the comfort of their own homes, eliminating the need for transportation and reducing wait times. It also makes it easier for individuals living in rural areas or those who have difficulty leaving their homes due to physical limitations or anxiety disorders to still receive quality care. Telemedicine has proven to be just as effective as traditional face-to-face therapy, making it a great option for those who need help but cannot access it due to geographical or financial constraints.

Another way technology is making mental healthcare more accessible is through apps and websites that offer self-guided care. These programs provide online tools and resources such as cognitive behavioral therapy (CBT), meditation exercises, and journaling activities that can help users manage their symptoms without having to leave the house or spend money on visit co-pays. This type of care can be especially beneficial for those dealing with depression, anxiety, or other mood disorders since they are able to receive treatment on their own time schedule without fear of judgment from others.

Technology is also being used to provide low-cost, private services such as online therapy. Sites like BetterHelp and TalkSpace offer individuals a chance to connect with licensed therapists without ever having to leave their homes. This type of service can be especially beneficial for those living in poverty or who otherwise cannot afford the high cost of traditional mental health care.

In addition, technology is helping to reduce the stigma associated with mental health within African American communities by providing appropriate education and resources about mental illness and treatment options. Websites such as MentalHealthAmerica.org and NAMI have developed programs specifically tailored toward addressing the unique challenges African Americans may face when it comes to seeking help for mental health conditions. Additionally, there are now social media campaigns designed to foster conversations about mental health and reduce the stigma associated with it.

In conclusion, technology is making a significant impact on how African Americans access mental health care. By utilizing telemedicine, self-guided care apps, and online therapy sites, individuals can receive quality treatment without having to worry about financial or geographic barriers. As more individuals become aware of these services, they may be more likely to take advantage of them in order to get the help they need. With the right support system in place, African American communities will be better equipped to recognize and address mental health issues among their members so that everyone can have access to proper care.

There are several strategies that can be implemented to improve access to mental health services for African Americans. From increasing funding for treatment to providing transportation options and reducing language barriers, there is much we can do to make sure everyone is able to get the care they need without facing discrimination or stigma. By creating a supportive environment in healthcare facilities, investing in technology-based solutions, and educating our communities about available resources, we can help ensure all individuals have access to quality mental healthcare regardless of their cultural background or economic circumstances. Now more than ever, it's time for us to come together and take action so that everyone would have the chance at a healthier, fulfilling life.

CHAPTER NINE

EXPLORING SELF-CARE AND COPING MECHANISMS FOR MENTAL HEALTH ISSUES

It's time to take a deep breath and look inward. In this chapter, we'll explore self-care practices and coping strategies that can help us manage our mental health symptoms, improve our overall well-being, and build resilience in the face of adversity. We'll discuss topics like mindfulness, journaling, yoga/meditation, support groups, exercise/dietary changes, and more.

It's important to remember that self-care is not selfish; it's a tool for navigating mental health issues with greater awareness and understanding. With thoughtful consideration of what works best for you, we can all learn effective coping strategies that bring us closer to our own healing and optimal well-being. So let's start the journey and learn some ways to explore self-care!

Self-care is the practice of taking care of your own physical, mental, and emotional needs. It's often seen as an essential part of managing mental health issues, as it can help to reduce stress, improve overall well-being, and build resilience in the face of adversity. Self-care takes many forms, and there is no one-size-fits-all approach. It's important to consider what unique needs you may have when exploring self-care and creating an individualized plan that works for you.

Self-care practices can range from simple activities like drinking a cup of tea or going for a walk to more complex strategies such as yoga or journaling. It can also include things like making dietary changes or reaching out to a support system for extra help. While these strategies are not "cures" for mental illness, they are effective tools that can help us to manage our symptoms and cope with difficult situations.

Taking time to invest in ourselves is an important part of self-care. It's easy to forget this when we're faced with the demands of everyday life, but it's important to remember that taking care of ourselves benefits both our mental and physical health. So set aside some time each day for activities that bring you joy and relaxation, and make sure to schedule regular check-ins with yourself on how you're feeling. With thoughtful consideration of what works best for you, we can all learn effective coping strategies that bring us closer to our own healing and optimal well-being.

Let's look at some of the self-care practices and coping strategies you can use to manage your mental health symptoms.

Mindfulness Practices

Mindfulness is a type of meditation that involves being fully present in the moment. It's based on the idea that focusing our attention on our current experience can help us to be more aware and attentive, both mentally and physically. Mindfulness practices can help us to recognize and accept difficult thoughts or feelings without judgment—something which can be particularly helpful when dealing with mental health issues.

Mindfulness exercises usually involve becoming aware of one's physical sensations, such as the breath, body movement, heart rate, temperature changes, etc., while also tuning into our thoughts and emotions. This practice helps to cultivate an attitude of non-judgmental acceptance toward whatever arises at the moment; it brings awareness to how we're feeling without getting caught up in the story.

Mindfulness can be practiced in a variety of ways. Some popular exercises include body scan meditation, mindful breathing, and loving-kindness meditation.

Body scan meditation is a mindfulness practice that involves systematically directing awareness to different parts of the body while noticing any sensations or emotions that may arise. It can be done either sitting or lying down and is often done in combination with deep breathing exercises.

The goal is to calmly observe each area of the body with the aim of noticing any physical sensations and mental states without judgment. This type of mindful awareness helps us to gain insight into how our bodies and minds interact and can be a powerful tool for managing difficult emotions.

When doing a body scan meditation, it's important to start at the feet and gradually move up toward the head. The idea is to pay attention to each part of the body, in turn relaxing any areas of tension as you go along. It's also helpful to use descriptive words as you scan through each area; for example, "warm," "tingly," "heavy," etc. As you become more comfortable with this practice, you may notice deeper subtleties, such as shifts in energy or emotion, that come with focusing on certain areas of your body.

Aside from helping us to better understand our physical and emotional selves, body scan meditation can also reduce stress levels and create a sense of calmness and inner peace. By taking time out from our busy lives to focus on the present moment without judgment or expectation, we can create an oasis of stillness even in times of difficulty and distress.

Mindful breathing, or mindful breathwork, is a type of mindfulness practice that involves focusing on the breath and how it moves through the body. This exercise can help to bring us back to the present moment and gain insight into our physical and emotional states. It can also help us to develop an attitude of non-judgmental acceptance toward whatever emotions may arise in the process.

When doing mindful breathing, it's important to focus on the breath without trying to control it. This means noticing how the inhalations and exhalations feel as they move in and out of your body—such as the sensation of air around your nose or chest expanding with each inhale. You can also observe any associated thoughts or emotions that may come up during this process. The goal is not to judge these experiences but rather observe them with curiosity and kindness.

It's also helpful to use visualizations when practicing mindful breathing; for example, imagining each breath flowing through your body like a wave or envisioning it filling you up with energy from head to toe. This helps you stay connected with your breath while developing an awareness of its impact throughout the body.

Mindful breathing can be practiced by both sitting and lying down; however, if you ever start feeling dizzy or uncomfortable while doing this exercise, take a break and refocus on something else until you're ready to continue again. It's important to remember that mindfulness practices are about being kind and patient with ourselves, so don't rush into anything before you're ready! With patience and dedication, we can all learn effective strategies that bring us closer to our own healing and optimal well-being.

Finally, loving-kindness meditation is a practice based on sending thoughts of kindness to ourselves and others—something which can be especially helpful for those dealing with mental health issues. This type of meditation involves repeating positive affirmations or phrases such as "May I be happy," "May I be free from suffering," and so on. The goal is to cultivate an attitude of loving-kindness toward ourselves and others while also becoming aware of any associated physical sensations or emotions that come up during the process.

This type of meditation encourages us to let go of judgment and criticism, allowing us to develop a more compassionate relationship with our inner experience. It can also help to reduce stress levels and promote feelings of acceptance and contentment, which are all important elements in managing mental health symptoms.

Overall, mindfulness practices offer a powerful tool for managing mental health issues. From body scan meditation and mindful breathing to loving kindness meditation, these strategies can help us to increase awareness of our physical and emotional selves while cultivating an attitude of non-judgmental acceptance toward whatever arises in the present moment. With thoughtful consideration of what works best for you, we can all learn effective coping strategies that bring us closer to our own healing and optimal well-being. So take some time today to explore what self-care can do for you!

Writing and Journaling

Writing and journaling are powerful tools for exploring our mental health issues and processing difficult emotions. By taking time to reflect on our thoughts and feelings, we can gain greater insight into ourselves while also developing a sense of clarity and peace of mind. This practice encourages us to let go of judgment and criticism, allowing us to become more compassionate with ourselves while building resilience in the face of adversity.

When it comes to writing and journaling, there are many approaches to choose from. It's important to consider what unique needs you may have when exploring what works best for you. Here are some popular methods:

Creative Writing - Creative writing is a way of exploring our inner world through the use of story-telling or creative expression. This type of writing can help us to express ourselves without worrying about grammar, spelling, or structure; it gives us permission to explore whatever ideas come up without judgment or criticism. This practice encourages us to recognize and accept our thoughts and feelings while also developing an attitude of self-compassion.

Journaling - Journaling is a great tool for processing difficult emotions in a non-judgmental way. It can be done in the form of a stream of conscious writing, where you simply write whatever comes to mind without worrying about structure or grammar, or it can involve a more structured approach, such as filling out a journaling prompt or making lists. The goal is to become aware of our thoughts and feelings without getting caught up in the story; this helps us to gain insight into ourselves while also learning how to manage our mental health symptoms with greater understanding and awareness.

Gratitude Journaling - Gratitude journaling is a great way to stay connected with the good things in our lives. This type of writing involves taking time each day to reflect on what we're thankful for; it encourages us to focus on the positive and cultivate an attitude of appreciation for even the small things that make life worth living. By practicing gratitude, not only do we become more mindful of our surroundings, but we also build resilience in the face of adversity and feel better overall.

For African Americans who are dealing with mental health issues, writing and journaling can be especially helpful. It allows them to express themselves without judgment or criticism while also developing an attitude of self-compassion and understanding. Writing can also help to reduce stress levels and promote feelings of acceptance, contentment, and peace of mind, which are all important elements in managing mental health symptoms.

Yoga

Yoga and meditation are powerful tools for managing mental health issues, as they help to reduce stress levels while also promoting feelings of acceptance and contentment. These practices can be especially helpful for African Americans dealing with mental health issues—not only do they offer a safe space to explore their inner world without judgment or criticism, but they can also build resilience in the face of adversity and cultivate an attitude of self-compassion.

Yoga is a physical practice that involves stretching, strengthening, and toning the body through various postures (asanas) combined with conscious breathing techniques (pranayama). This type of exercise can help to improve physical and mental well-being, as it encourages us to become aware of our bodies in a non-judgmental way while also increasing our flexibility and strength.

By exploring different postures of yoga, we can learn effective strategies that bring us closer to our own healing and optimal well-being. Not only do these practices help us become more mindful of our bodies in a non-judgmental way, but they also help us build strength physically and mentally! So next time you need some extra love & attention, try experimenting with one (or all!) of these postures & see how they make you feel!

Yoga also offers many psychological benefits for those dealing with mental health issues. It helps to reduce stress and anxiety levels while promoting feelings of acceptance, contentment, and peace of mind. It encourages us to develop an attitude of self-compassion as we become aware of our own thoughts and emotions without judgment or criticism. This type of mindful awareness can be especially helpful for African Americans who are struggling with mental health issues, as it allows them to explore their inner world in a safe space while building resilience in the face of adversity.

For those new to yoga, it's important to start slowly and honor your own pace. It can also be helpful to find a qualified instructor who can guide you through the postures while ensuring that you're doing them safely and correctly. Additionally, there are many online resources available for people looking for yoga instruction—video tutorials, audio recordings of guided practices, etc. No matter how you choose to practice Yoga, it's important to remember that this is an individual journey—so take some time today to explore what works best for you!

Exercise

Exercise is an important part of maintaining physical health and well-being, as it helps to improve cardiovascular fitness while also strengthening bones and muscles. It can also be a powerful tool for managing mental health issues—not only does it reduce stress levels, but it also promotes feelings of acceptance, contentment, and peace of mind. This makes exercise especially helpful for African Americans who are dealing with mental health issues, as it allows them to explore their inner world without judgment or criticism while also building resilience in the face of adversity.

When it comes to exercise, there are many approaches to choose from—so take some time today to explore what works best for you! Here are some popular methods:

Aerobic Exercise – Aerobic exercise, also known as "cardio," is a type of physical activity that increases heart rate and breathing while also improving overall fitness. This can include activities such as walking, jogging, swimming, biking, dancing, or any other activity that gets your heart rate up. Not only does this type of exercise help to reduce stress levels, but it also promotes feelings of acceptance and contentment while helping to increase self-confidence in the process.

Strength Training – Strength training is another popular form of exercise that helps to build muscle strength and improve bone density. This can include activities such as weightlifting or bodyweight exercises such as push-ups, squats, and sit-ups. Not only does this type of exercise help to improve physical well-being, but it can also be a powerful tool for managing mental health issues. It encourages us to become aware of our bodies in a non-judgmental way while also building resilience in the face of adversity.

Flexibility Training – Flexibility training is a type of exercise that helps to improve joint mobility and range of motion. This can include activities such as stretching, yoga, or Pilates. Not only does this type of exercise help to reduce stress levels, but it also encourages us to become aware of our bodies in a non-judgmental way while cultivating an attitude of self-compassion and understanding. This makes flexibility training especially helpful for African Americans who are dealing with mental health issues, as it allows them to explore their inner world in a safe space while building resilience in the face of adversity.

No matter what type of exercise you choose to do, it's important to make sure that you're doing it safely. This means taking breaks when needed and listening to your body so that you don't overdo it. Additionally, if you ever start feeling dizzy or uncomfortable while exercising, take a break and refocus on something else until you're ready to continue again. It's also helpful to consult with a qualified health professional who can provide advice about which types of exercises are best suited for your individual needs.

Exercise can also be a great way to connect with other people. Joining an exercise group, or even just exercising with a friend, can help add structure and accountability to your fitness routine while also providing social support—something which is especially important for those dealing with mental health issues. It's also helpful to look into local resources such as community centers or organizations that offer classes or workshops related to physical activity. This can provide an opportunity for African Americans who are dealing with mental health issues to explore their inner world in a safe space while building resilience in the face of adversity.

Don't forget that there's no "one size fits all" approach when it comes to exercise! What works best for one person may not necessarily work for another, so remember to take some time today to explore what works best for your individual needs and interests. Additionally, there are many online resources available if you need extra motivation or guidance on how to structure your exercise routine, so don't hesitate to look into these as well!

Finally, it's important to remember that exercise is just one way to manage mental health issues, so take some time today to explore other strategies as well. This could include things like writing and journaling, yoga and meditation, mindfulness techniques, or any other activity that helps you to build resilience in the face of adversity. By taking a holistic approach to managing mental health symptoms, we can become more compassionate with ourselves while also gaining insight into our own thoughts and emotions in a safe space.

Dietary Changes

Dietary changes can play an important role in managing mental health issues, as they can help to reduce stress levels while also improving overall physical and mental well-being. This makes it especially important for African American communities to pay attention to what they eat, as the stigma of mental health issues can often lead people in these communities to put their own health and well-being on the back burner.

The first step in making dietary changes is to identify any unhealthy eating habits or patterns that may be contributing to mental health issues. This could include anything from regularly consuming high-sugar or processed foods, skipping meals, or even not getting enough good-quality food each day. Once any unhealthy habits are identified, it's important to make a plan for changing them.

Replacing sugary drinks with water and adding more fruits and vegetables into the diet should be top priorities when it comes to making dietary changes. Filling up with nutrient-rich plants can help the body and mind feel better, as these foods are packed with important vitamins and minerals that can support overall physical health.

It's also a good idea to limit or avoid processed foods whenever possible, as these are often high in unhealthy fats and sugars. These types of food can cause blood sugar levels to spike, which can lead to a crash later on and even contribute to feelings of irritability or sadness. Instead, focus on whole, unprocessed options like nuts, seeds, legumes, and whole grains.

Including healthy fats in the diet is important too. Healthy sources of fat like avocados, salmon, olive oil, chia seeds, and walnuts all contain essential fatty acids that can help the body and brain function optimally. Eating these types of fats can also help to reduce any inflammation in the body, which can have a positive impact on mood.

Making sure to get enough protein in the diet is important too. Protein provides essential amino acids that help the body produce neurotransmitters that regulate mood and energy levels, so getting adequate amounts each day is key. Good sources of plant-based proteins include nuts and seeds, legumes like beans, lentils, and chickpeas, and whole grains such as quinoa and brown rice.

It's important to be mindful when it comes to eating. Eating slowly and paying attention to hunger cues rather than eating on autopilot can help to support a healthy relationship with food. This is especially important for African American communities, as there can be additional pressures and stigma associated with being overweight or obese, which can add to the stress of managing mental health issues.

Making dietary changes isn't always easy, so it's important to be patient and work on making small steps toward better nutrition each day. It may also be helpful to seek out professional guidance from a registered dietitian or nutritionist who can provide tailored advice and support based on individual needs.

Dietary changes are just one part of managing mental health issues, but they can play an important role in overall well-being. Making sure to get enough good-quality, nutrient-rich food each day can help to reduce stress levels and improve physical and mental health, which is essential for African Americans who are often dealing with the additional burden of the stigma associated with mental health issues. With a little bit of effort, it's possible to make dietary changes that will have a positive impact on overall mental health.

Practicing Self-Compassion

Self-compassion is an important component of managing mental health issues, and it's especially important for African Americans who often deal with the additional burden of stigma associated with mental health concerns. Self-compassion involves cultivating a kind and understanding attitude toward oneself, even when faced with difficult emotions or challenging situations. It's an invaluable tool for people struggling with mental health issues because it can help to reduce feelings of shame or guilt while also empowering individuals to take control over their own healing process.

The first step in practicing self-compassion is to recognize and acknowledge difficult feelings. Often, people in the African American community are made to feel ashamed of their emotions or thoughts, which can lead them to attempt to ignore or deny what they're feeling. This can be damaging for long-term mental health, as not addressing these issues can cause them to fester and become worse over time. Acknowledging and allowing yourself to experience whatever you're feeling can help to reduce any shame associated with these emotions while also helping to address the root causes of your mental health concerns.

The next step is learning how to respond kindly and compassionately when faced with difficult feelings or situations. Instead of getting angry with yourself or being overly critical, try responding as if talking to a close friend or loved one. This could involve speaking kindly and offering words of encouragement, as well as recognizing that it's okay to make mistakes and not be perfect all the time. Practicing self-compassion can also help to reduce any feelings of stress or anxiety associated with mental health issues by providing comfort and assurance in times of need.

It's important to remember that self-compassion is an ongoing process, and it's something that needs to be practiced regularly for it to have the most benefit. In order to nurture this attitude of kindness toward yourself, take some time each day to engage in activities that you find calming or enjoyable, such as reading, going for a walk, or listening to music. Taking some time each day to focus on self-care can help to reduce stress levels and improve your overall mental health.

Finally, it's important to recognize that practicing self-compassion is not a sign of weakness or giving up; rather, it's an act of strength that shows that you care about yourself and are actively working toward improving your well-being. It can also be beneficial to seek out support from friends and family who can provide emotional understanding when needed.

At the end of the day, self-care and coping mechanisms can be powerful tools for managing mental health issues in the African American community. By engaging in activities that promote physical and mental well-being, developing healthy eating habits, and practicing self-compassion, we can build resilience in the face of adversity while also reducing feelings of the stigma associated with mental health concerns. With a little bit of effort, it's possible to make changes that will have a positive impact on overall mental health—so take some time today to explore which strategies work best for you!

CHAPTER TEN

FAITH-BASED APPROACHES TO MENTAL HEALTH

In African-American communities, faith-based approaches to mental health can provide invaluable support and resources for individuals coping with a mental disorder. Religion can offer guidance on how to cope with the pain, anguish, and stigma associated with a mental illness. And it provides an opportunity for people to connect on a spiritual level and receive comfort from their peers in the community.

This chapter will take a look at how faith-based approaches can be used as part of treatment plans for those suffering from mental illnesses. We'll explore ways that spiritual practices such as prayer and meditation can help manage symptoms, religious counseling techniques that may be beneficial, and community outreach programs designed specifically to address issues surrounding mental health in African American communities. So let's dive in and learn more about how faith-based approaches can make a difference for those struggling with mental health issues.

Prayer and Other Religious Practices

Prayer and other religious practices have been used by African Americans for centuries as a way to cope with mental illness. Prayer can provide comfort, strength, and guidance in difficult times and is often seen as an integral part of the healing process. Studies have also shown that engaging in spiritual practices such as prayer can help reduce symptoms of depression, anxiety, stress, and post-traumatic stress disorder (PTSD).

Prayer is often seen as a way to connect with a higher power, whether it be God, an ancestor, or the universe. It can provide comfort and support in times of distress and can help individuals find peace and solace in moments of turmoil. Prayer can enable African Americans to experience a sense of belonging, connectedness, and hope—something that is often lacking when dealing with mental health issues. For many individuals, prayer can be used as a form of self-care—a way to take care of oneself spiritually during difficult times.

In addition to prayer, there are other religious practices that may be beneficial for those suffering from mental illness.

Meditation has been found to reduce anxiety levels and improve overall well-being by helping individuals to refocus their thoughts and put them into perspective. Participating in religious services or attending weekly church groups can provide a sense of community, acceptance, and support from peers, which can be an important component of recovery for many. Finally, engaging in activities such as writing inspirational scriptures or quotes on paper or taking part in creative projects like painting or drawing can help to manifest positive thoughts and feelings.

When it comes to choosing the right approach for managing mental health issues through faith-based practices, it's important to consider the individual needs of each person. Some may find comfort in prayer, while others may benefit more from meditation or participating in religious services. It's also important to remember that not all faith-based approaches will be helpful for everyone. It's best to consult a mental health professional for guidance on which approaches will be the most beneficial for each individual.

It's important to remember that while faith-based practices can be a great tool in managing symptoms of mental illness, they should not be used as a substitute for proper medical care. Consulting with a licensed therapist or psychiatrist is essential when dealing with any form of mental illness and should always come first before exploring different spiritual solutions.

Faith-based community outreach programs tailored specifically to address the stigma surrounding mental health in African American communities have become increasingly popular over the years. These programs may focus on providing education on recognizing signs of a mental illness or promoting support groups for individuals who are struggling. Community outreach programs often provide valuable resources such as access to mental health professionals, support groups, and spiritual guidance.

The stigma surrounding mental health in African American communities is an important issue that must be addressed through education, awareness, and compassion. Faith-based approaches can provide invaluable assistance in aiding individuals who are struggling with mental illness by offering comfort, support, guidance, and connection to the community. By exploring different spiritual practices and working with religious counselors, those dealing with mental health issues can find ways to cope with symptoms while embracing their belief systems.

Religious Counseling for Mental Health Issues

Religious counseling has become an increasingly popular form of therapy when it comes to managing mental health issues in the African American community. This type of counseling focuses on utilizing religious texts, scriptures, and teachings as a source of support and guidance for individuals with mental illness. It can be an effective approach for those who are deeply rooted in their faith and seek spiritual guidance during difficult times.

During religious counseling sessions, counselors will often use scripture to provide comfort and hope while also offering practical advice about how to cope with symptoms or external stressors that may be causing distress. Discussions may cover topics such as forgiveness, grace, and mercy while exploring the idea of a higher power. It is important to note that religious counseling does not replace professional therapy—it can be used as an adjunct or supplemental form of treatment for those seeking spiritual guidance.

Religious counselors are typically well-versed in various faiths and denominations, enabling them to provide clients with individualized guidance based on their beliefs. This allows them to make meaningful connections between faith and mental health issues, bridging the gap between traditional therapy models and spiritual practices. Furthermore, they can help individuals find deeper meaning within their own lives by exploring questions related to one's purpose or calling in life.

When it comes to addressing topics such as forgiveness or grace during counseling sessions, religious counselors can help provide clarity and understanding. They can explore how the concepts of grace and forgiveness are rooted in various religious texts, offering insight and guidance for individuals seeking spiritual support. This type of counseling is beneficial for those who want to reconcile their faith with their mental health issues or seek solace from a higher power during difficult times.

Another important aspect of religious counseling is helping individuals find ways to connect with their faith community. Counselors can assist clients in finding local churches, temples, mosques, or other places of worship that may be able to offer support. There are numerous organizations and programs available that specialize in providing religious-based services, such as stress management classes, coping strategies workshops, group therapy sessions, and more. These services are often tailored specifically to address the needs of African-Americans struggling with mental health issues.

Religious counseling provides valuable support and guidance for those dealing with mental health issues in the African American community. It offers individuals an opportunity to explore questions related to their faith while receiving support and understanding from a spiritual perspective. Religious counselors can provide insight into the various aspects of faith while helping individuals reconcile their beliefs with their mental illness. This type of counseling can be a powerful tool for those looking to find hope and solace during difficult times.

How Churches Can Play a Part in Improving Access to Care

Churches play an integral role in providing spiritual support and guidance to individuals with mental illnesses, but they can also be a valuable resource for improving access to care within the African American community. Research shows that African Americans are more likely to seek help from religious institutions than from medical professionals, making it essential for churches to become knowledgeable about mental health and create an environment where individuals feel comfortable discussing such issues.

Churches can start by addressing the stigmas surrounding mental illness in their communities. By having an open dialogue on the subject and encouraging individuals to discuss their feelings with their peers or clergy members, members of the congregation will begin to normalize conversations about mental health and reduce any fear associated with seeking help. As these conversations take place, churches can also disseminate information on available resources and encourage people to connect with other community-based organizations that specialize in providing services for individuals struggling with mental health issues.

In addition, churches can advocate resources and funding to improve access to mental health care. By connecting with elected officials and other professionals in the community, they can work to increase funding for mental health programs, make sure existing programs are adequately staffed, and provide additional educational programs that teach people about different types of illnesses and treatments available. This type of advocacy is especially important because African Americans often lack access to adequate healthcare due to economic or geographical barriers.

Churches can also lend a hand by offering support groups for individuals struggling with mental illness. Such groups may be led by clergy members, counselors, or trained volunteers who can listen without judgment and provide assistance in navigating treatment options or helping them find resources. These support groups offer a safe space where individuals feel heard and understood rather than judged or shamed.

Finally, churches can also provide education about mental health issues. By hosting seminars and workshops on topics such as depression, anxiety, and suicide prevention, members of the congregation can begin to understand the signs and symptoms associated with different illnesses and learn tools for coping or providing assistance to loved ones. Additionally, churches can partner with medical professionals in the community so that they can refer people who need additional help to appropriate resources.

Overcoming Obstacles in Implementing Faith-Based Practices

In order to reduce the stigma of mental health within the African American community, one approach that has proven successful is utilizing faith-based practices. Faith-based approaches focus on bringing together spiritual and psychological healing techniques to help people who suffer from mental illness. However, there are many obstacles involved in implementing these practices in a way that proves effective for the mentally ill individual. By understanding and recognizing these challenges, we can better equip ourselves with the knowledge and resources necessary to overcome them.

The first obstacle to implementing faith-based practices is perhaps one of the most challenging: overcoming skepticism and negative attitudes toward faith-based therapies among individuals within the African American community. For some, traditional religious beliefs can make them wary of incorporating psychological care into religious practices. It is important to create an open dialogue between individuals and their pastors or other faith-based leaders in order to bridge the gap between spiritual and psychological healing.

A second obstacle to implementing faith-based practices is the lack of resources available. Many churches and other religious settings don't have the material resources or the professional training necessary for effective mental health care. This can be a deterrent to those who are seeking help but may not have access to more comprehensive mental health services. To combat this, community members should work together to create education programs that provide information about mental health, as well as programs that provide support and guidance for individuals who seek out psychotherapy in their spiritual contexts.

A third obstacle to implementing faith-based practices within African American communities is the lack of mental health professionals who are knowledgeable and willing to work with individuals in a spiritual context. Mental health professionals should be trained on how to integrate spiritual healing into their psychological care so that they can better understand and meet the needs of their clients. It is also important for these mental health professionals to have adequate resources available in order for them to provide effective treatment.

Finally, it can be difficult for some people in the African American community to access faith-based treatments because of cultural differences between different churches or denominations. While many religious organizations are eager to help those suffering from mental illness, there may still be issues related to language barriers or a lack of understanding of different cultural beliefs and values. It is important that individuals are able to access a variety of faith-based treatments so that they can find an approach that works best for them.

By working together, we can reduce the stigma of mental health in the African American community and provide a safe and supportive environment for those who are suffering from mental illness. By providing education programs about mental health issues, as well as resources for faith-based treatments, we can help ensure that individuals have access to the care they need. We must also recognize the challenges related to utilizing faith-based approaches in order to better equip ourselves with the knowledge and resources necessary for effective psychological and spiritual healing. Together, we can work toward creating an open dialogue where all people feel supported when seeking out mental health treatment.

CHAPTER ELEVEN
UPLIFTING STORIES OF AFRICAN AMERICAN MENTAL HEALTH ADVOCATES

This chapter is dedicated to the brave African American mental health advocates who have taken their struggles and forged them into a force of good. Their stories are powerful examples of resilience, strength, and courage in the face of adversity.

From activists raising awareness about mental health issues to those opening up dialogues about getting professional help, these individuals serve as shining beacons of hope. They are a reminder that no matter how dark things may seem, it's always possible to find light at the end of the tunnel. Their inspiring stories will surely touch our hearts and remind us that there's always something we can do to make a difference in our own lives and those around us. Let's take a look!

The Story of Taraji P. Henson

The Story of Taraji P. Henson is one of hope and resilience in the face of adversity. As an actress, producer, and founder of the Boris Lawrence Henson Foundation, she has proven to be an advocate for mental health awareness within the African American community.

Taraji P. Henson has openly discussed her struggles with anxiety and depression, making it a point to speak up on the importance of getting professional help for one's mental health. With that in mind, she founded the Boris Lawrence Henson Foundation in 2018 to provide much-needed resources and support for people dealing with mental illness in the African American community. This is especially important since there are still numerous stigmas and barriers to accessing mental health care within this population.

Through her foundation, Taraji P. Henson has spearheaded initiatives such as free therapy sessions, funding scholarships for African American students wanting to pursue careers in the field of mental health, and launching "Peace of Mind with Taraji" on Facebook. This program offers viewers the opportunity to learn more about mental health, see a real-time therapy session in action, and hear first-hand stories from celebrities who have dealt with similar issues.

In addition to her foundation work, Taraji P. Henson has also been featured in various magazines, discussing the importance of self-care and advocating for mental wellness within the African American community. The impact of Taraji P. Henson's advocacy is undeniable. By speaking openly about her own struggles with mental health, she has brought much-needed attention to the issue within the African American community and inspired countless people to seek help for themselves or be there for someone else who needs support.

The story of Taraji P. Henson is a powerful reminder that no matter what kind of adversity we face, it's always possible to overcome our struggles and make a difference in the lives of others. Thanks to her tireless advocacy work, she has opened up dialogues about mental health and provided valuable resources for those who need them. She truly serves as an inspiring example of hope and resilience in times of difficulty. Let us continue to be empowered by her success story and strive to create a world where everyone can get the help they need regardless of their race or ethnicity.

Charlamagne Tha God

Charlamagne Tha God is an influential radio personality, author, and mental health advocate who has made a huge impact on the African American community. His story of resilience and determination in the face of adversity is inspiring and uplifting.

Born in South Carolina in 1978, Charlamagne Tha God has become a household name through his career in radio and his highly popular podcast "The Breakfast Club." His show features an array of celebrities and notable figures discussing social issues, pop culture topics, and more.

In addition to his work on the airwaves, Charlamagne Tha God is also an advocate for mental health awareness within the African American community. After battling depression and anxiety himself, he has made it a point to speak up about the importance of getting professional help when dealing with mental health problems. Through interviews, events, and books such as *Shook One: Anxiety Playing Tricks On Me* and his Mental Wealth Alliance charity, he has helped to raise awareness of mental health issues in the Black community and to break down the stigma associated with mental illness.

Tha God's advocacy work is important because it addresses a number of unique challenges that African Americans face when it comes to mental health. These include the lack of access to resources, the impact of racism and discrimination on Black mental health, and the stigma associated with seeking help for one's struggles. Through Mental Wealth Alliance (MWA), Charlamagne Tha God has provided free therapy sessions for ten million Black Americans over the next five years as well as training and resources to increase the number of qualified Black mental health professionals. His efforts have also helped to open up dialogues about mental health and to make it more acceptable to seek help for these issues.

Charlamagne Tha God's story is a powerful reminder that no matter what kind of adversity we face, it's always possible to overcome our struggles and make a difference in the lives of others. By speaking openly about his own struggles with mental health, he has raised awareness and inspired countless people to seek help or support someone else who needs it. His tireless advocacy work has shown us that there is always something we can do to create a world where everyone can get the help they need regardless of their race or ethnicity.

Let us be motivated by his story and continue to stand up for mental health awareness on a global level. Here's to Charlamagne Tha God!

Joy Harden Bradford

Joy Harden Bradford is an incredible mental health advocate who is making a huge impact on the African American community. Through her weekly podcast, Therapy for Black Girls, speaking engagements around the country, online courses, and individual therapy sessions, she has provided invaluable resources and support to help Black women overcome the unique challenges they face in terms of mental health.

Each week, the Therapy for Black Girls podcast features interviews with experts and personal stories from Black women who are struggling with mental health issues. Through these conversations, Bradford provides practical advice on how to manage stress, build healthy relationships, and improve overall mental wellness. She also offers workshops and training for professionals who work with Black women to help them better understand their unique needs when it comes to mental health.

In addition to her podcast, Bradford also offers online courses on topics such as stress management, anxiety, and self-care. These courses are designed to help Black women develop the skills they need to effectively manage their mental health issues and improve overall well-being. She also provides individual therapy sessions for Black women who are struggling with mental health problems, offering a safe space where they can talk about their experiences without fear of judgment or stigma.

Bradford's services are invaluable in helping to break down the barriers that African Americans face when it comes to accessing mental healthcare. Through her work, she has opened up conversations about mental health within the Black community and made it more acceptable for people to seek professional help for their struggles. Her efforts have also provided much-needed resources and support for those who need it, helping to reduce the stigma associated with seeking help and making mental health care more accessible.

Bradford's story is one of resilience and determination in the face of adversity. Her work has shown us that no matter what kind of obstacles we may face, it's always possible to make a difference in the lives of others. Thanks to her tireless advocacy work, she has opened up dialogues about mental health within the African American community and inspired countless people to seek help or be there for someone else who needs support.

As we have seen, these inspiring African American mental health advocates are true beacons of hope. Through their stories of resilience and determination in the face of adversity, they have opened up conversations about mental health within the Black community and provided much-needed resources for those who need them. They serve as a reminder that no matter how dark things may seem, there is always something we can do to make a difference in our own lives and those around us. Let us continue to be empowered by their stories and strive to create a world where everyone can get the help they need regardless of their race or ethnicity. Here's to uplifting stories of African American mental health advocates!

CHAPTER TWELVE
MOVING FORWARD WITH MENTAL HEALTH CARE IN AFRICAN AMERICAN COMMUNITY

The world is full of judgment and stigma, especially when it comes to mental health care in African American communities. We have come a long way since the days of not understanding or taking depression and other mental illnesses seriously. But there's still so much more work to be done for us to move forward and create an inclusive atmosphere that understands and accepts mental illness.

In this chapter, we will examine how far we've come with tackling the stigma around mental health care in African American communities, as well as what needs to be done to continue making progress. We'll talk about media representation, bias toward certain groups, and how to create an environment that promotes understanding instead of judgment and discrimination. It's time for us all to move forward together in creating a more inclusive and understanding future. Let's get started!

Positive Representation in the Media: A Step in the Right Direction

It's no surprise that media representation of mental health issues has been incredibly lacking—particularly when it comes to African American communities. The stigma surrounding mental illness can be heavily perpetuated by the way it is portrayed in the media, with many narratives focusing on only the negative aspects rather than highlighting any potential solutions or positive steps being taken.

Thankfully, we are beginning to see more and more positive representations of mental health care in African American communities in the media. Whether it's films, television shows, YouTube videos, or podcasts, there is a growing number of stories that focus on the importance of seeking out professional help and destigmatizing mental illness. This is an incredibly powerful step in the right direction for our society as a whole.

By highlighting these positive stories, we can start to break down the stigma and create an environment that is more understanding and supportive of those suffering from mental health issues. Not only does this help to create a safe and inviting atmosphere for anyone who needs help, but it also serves as an example of what could be—showing others that it's okay to seek out mental health care, even if they come from a traditionally marginalized community.

Of course, there are still plenty of negative representations in the media when it comes to mental health care in African American communities. These range from damaging stereotypes about Black people being "lazy" or "crazy" to narratives that suggest all Black people have the same experience with depression or anxiety.

It's important to recognize these damaging portrayals and speak out against them. We need to be proactive in challenging the stereotypes and discrimination that can still exist within certain media representations of mental health care. By doing so, we can help create an environment that is more accepting and understanding—one where everyone feels safe seeking out help, regardless of their background or ethnicity.

Ultimately, positive representation of mental health care in African American communities is an important first step in tackling the stigma and discrimination that still exists within our society. We need to continue to push forward with creating more inclusive media narratives and challenging any damaging stereotypes that are still present. With continued progress, we can create a world where everyone feels comfortable taking the steps they need to get the help they deserve. Let's work together to make this happen!

Accessibility to Quality Care: Creating an Inclusive Environment

When it comes to mental health care, accessibility is key—especially for those in traditionally marginalized communities such as African Americans. Unfortunately, many individuals are still struggling to gain access to quality mental health care. Whether it's due to cost, a lack of information about services available, or existing biases against certain groups, the reality is that too many people are being left behind when it comes to receiving the help they need.

It's time for us to create an environment that is more inclusive and understanding of all people seeking out mental health care, regardless of their background. This means ensuring everyone has equal access to quality services, as well as providing the resources and support necessary for those who need it.

One way to do this is by working to provide more affordable options for mental health care. This includes both creating more affordable private services as well as expanding public programs, such as Medicaid. This will help individuals who may not be able to afford traditional services access the care they need without having to worry about financial burdens.

Another important step is making sure everyone has access to information about available mental health services—particularly in African American communities, where there can often be a lack of knowledge or understanding about what's out there. We need to create more accessible and comprehensive resources that people can easily find, including online resources on websites and social media platforms.

Finally, it's essential to address existing biases that can prevent people from seeking out mental health care. This includes working with mental health professionals to ensure they are actively challenging their own implicit biases and providing culturally competent care. It also means fostering an environment that is more accepting of individuals who may feel uncomfortable or judged when discussing mental illness.

By taking these steps, we can create a world where everyone has access to the quality mental health care they deserve—no matter what their background or ethnicity is. It's time for us all to move forward together in creating a more inclusive and understanding future for those suffering from mental health conditions.

Taking Action Together for a Brighter Future

When it comes to tackling the stigma around mental health care in African American communities, we all have a role to play. From those who are actively seeking out help for their own mental health issues to allies speaking up against discrimination or supporting friends and family members who are facing struggles—we can all take action together for a brighter future for our communities.

One of the most important steps we can take is to be open and honest about our own experiences with mental illness. We must break down the stigma around discussing mental health issues by sharing our stories and supporting one another in a respectful and non-judgmental way. This helps to create an environment where individuals feel comfortable seeking out help without fear of judgment or discrimination.

We also need to challenge any existing stereotypes or biased narratives surrounding mental illness. Whether it's in the media or in conversations with family and friends, it's essential to speak up against any damaging representations that may still exist. We can do this by speaking out against incorrect assumptions, challenging bias when we hear it, and celebrating positive stories that are showing progress toward destigmatizing mental health care.

It's also important to take action from a policy standpoint, supporting initiatives such as making mental health services more affordable and accessible, as well as promoting education about the importance of seeking help when needed. By advocating for change on this level, we can create an environment that is more supportive and understanding of individuals who need help.

Finally, it's essential to support local organizations that are dedicated to providing quality mental health care to underserved communities. This could include donating money or volunteering time—anything you can do to increase awareness and access to these vital services.

By taking these steps together, we can create a brighter future for all those struggling with mental illness in African American communities. It's time for us all to step up and create an environment that is more inclusive and understanding of mental health issues. Let's work together to make this happen!

Conclusion

The stigma surrounding mental health in the African American community is real and pervasive, yet it doesn't have to be that way. By educating ourselves on mental health issues, understanding our cultural norms and attitudes, creating supportive networks in our communities, and advocating for better access to care, we can create a brighter future for those struggling with mental illness.

This book has explored how the stigma of mental health in the African American community affects individuals and families. From recognizing symptoms of mental illness to accessing quality care and overcoming stigmas associated with seeking help, this book seeks to empower its readers so they can take control of their own mental well-being.

This book has further discussed why this stigma exists and how it can be overcome, as well as providing knowledge and resources for improving mental health. It has also highlighted stories of those who have experienced the stigma and shown how they have worked through it to get help.

The key takeaways of this book are that it is important to recognize the stigma of mental health in African American communities and to understand why it exists. It is also essential to be aware of various cultural norms, family dynamics, religious beliefs, and traditions that can influence how mental health is viewed and treated. Additionally, we should advocate better access to care in order to ensure everyone has access to quality mental health services.

We must also strive to educate ourselves and our communities on mental illness so that we can create more inclusive representation and understanding. It is also important to foster a supportive environment for those living with mental illness by providing resources such as self-care practices, faith-based approaches, healing practices, support groups, and peer-to-peer counseling.

It is also important to celebrate the successes of those who have overcome their mental health struggles and become advocates for others in similar situations. Finally, we must recognize that mental health is a universal issue and not something to be ashamed of or ignored.

Seeking help for mental health issues is an important step that should not be overlooked or ignored. It can be difficult to ask for help, but it is essential if we want to improve our overall well-being. When we seek help, we are taking charge of our own well-being and showing ourselves that we care enough to make a positive change.

There are many ways to get help, including talking with a therapist or counselor, joining a support group, using self-care practices such as yoga or meditation, and connecting with family and friends who can provide emotional support. We must also strive to find quality mental healthcare in our communities by understanding our rights when it comes to accessing care and advocating for better resources.

It is important to remember that mental health issues affect everyone at some point in their lives, and it's okay to ask for help. Seeking help does not have to be daunting or shameful; it can be a positive experience that leads to improved mental well-being.

There are many famous sayings on the importance of mental health and seeking help, such as "We all need someone to talk to" by Maya Angelou and "It does not matter how slowly you go as long as you do not stop" by Confucius. Sayings like these can be helpful in understanding that emotional challenges are normal and that we are not alone in our struggles.

"The most beautiful people we have known are those who have known defeat, known suffering, known struggle, known loss, and have found their way out of the depths," by Elisabeth Kübler-Ross, is a reminder that strength can be found even in the darkest times.

"You can't always control what goes on outside. But you can always control what goes on inside," by Wayne Dyer, is a reminder of the power of self-care.

In conclusion, this book has shown how we can create a brighter future for those living with mental illness by recognizing the stigma of mental health in African American communities and taking steps to break it down. We must strive to provide quality care, understand cultural norms, find support networks, and celebrate successes. It is only through education, advocacy, and support that we can make real progress in improving mental health in African American communities.

Thank you for reading this book. We hope it has empowered you to take control of your mental well-being and made you more aware of the stigma surrounding mental health in African American communities. Together, we can create a healthier future for everyone.

Glossary

Anxiety Disorders: Anxiety disorders are mental health conditions characterized by excessive fear, worry, and unease in response to a perceived threat. Common anxiety disorders include panic disorder, phobias, social anxiety disorder, obsessive-compulsive disorder (OCD), generalized anxiety disorder (GAD), and post-traumatic stress disorder (PTSD).

Depression: Depression is a mental health disorder characterized by persistent feelings of sadness, loss of interest in activities, difficulty sleeping or eating, fatigue, and impaired concentration. It is the most common mental illness among adults in the United States.

Bipolar Disorder: Bipolar disorder is a mental health condition characterized by extreme mood swings between periods of mania (high energy and euphoria) and depression (low energy and hopelessness). It is sometimes referred to as manic-depressive disorder.

Schizophrenia: Schizophrenia is a serious mental health disorder characterized by disturbances in thought processes, behavior, and perceptions. Symptoms can include hallucinations, delusions, disorganized thinking or speech, loss of motivation, impaired social functioning, and withdrawal from society.

Post-Traumatic Stress Disorder (PTSD): PTSD is a mental health condition triggered by a traumatic event in which the individual experiences flashbacks, nightmares, and intrusive thoughts related to the event. Symptoms can include anxiety, insomnia, difficulty concentrating, irritability or anger outbursts, and avoidance of activities or situations that remind them of the trauma.

Substance Abuse: Substance abuse is defined as the excessive or problematic use of drugs or alcohol which can lead to physical and psychological dependence. It includes illicit substances as well as prescription drugs when used for non-medical purposes.

Mental Health Stigma: Mental health stigma is defined as negative attitudes and beliefs about mental illness that can lead to discrimination and isolation from society. While these attitudes vary based on cultural norms, they are often rooted in fear or misunderstanding of the condition.

Cultural Competency: Cultural competency refers to the ability to interact effectively and respectfully with people from different cultures in order to provide quality care tailored to their unique cultural needs. It involves being able to recognize, understand, and address cultural differences in healthcare settings while remaining respectful of individuals' cultural backgrounds.

Cultural Norms: Cultural norms refer to shared values, beliefs, and behavior shared by a particular group of people. They can include language, clothing, food preferences, attitudes toward health and wellness, religious or spiritual beliefs, and more.

Therapy: Therapy is the process of talking with a trained professional about feelings, thoughts, and experiences in order to gain insight into and overcome emotional or behavioral problems. It can take many forms, including individual therapy, couples counseling, family therapy, art therapy, play therapy, etc.

Self-Care: Self-care refers to taking intentional steps to prioritize one's physical, emotional, and psychological well-being in order to maintain and improve overall health. This can involve establishing healthy routines such as getting enough sleep and eating nutritious meals, as well as engaging in activities that bring pleasure and relaxation.

Coping Mechanisms: Coping mechanisms are strategies used to manage difficult feelings or situations. Common coping strategies include talking to a friend, journaling, reading, exercising, listening to music, spending time outdoors, and more.

Mindfulness: Mindfulness is a mental state achieved by focusing one's attention on the present moment without judgment. It can help reduce stress and increase awareness of physical sensations and thoughts, allowing for greater self-regulation.

Journaling: Journaling is the practice of writing down thoughts, feelings, and experiences in order to gain clarity or understanding. This can be helpful for individuals who find it difficult to verbalize their emotions or who want to explore their innermost thoughts in a safe and non-judgmental space.

Yoga: Yoga is an ancient practice that includes physical postures, breathing exercises, and meditation designed to relax the body and mind. It can help improve flexibility, reduce stress, and increase strength.

Support Group: A support group is a gathering of individuals who come together to share their experiences and provide emotional support to one another. They often focus on specific topics such as addiction recovery or grief counseling.

Prayer: Prayer is a spiritual practice of communication with a higher power. It involves talking directly to God or another deity in order to express gratitude, ask for guidance, receive blessings, etc.

Meditation: Meditation is a practice of self-reflection and mental discipline that can help to reduce stress and improve clarity of thought. It involves focusing on the breath or repeating a phrase to achieve a sense of calmness and inner peace.

Religious Counseling: Religious counseling is therapy in which the practitioner focuses on the individual's religious beliefs and practices as part of their treatment plan. This may include exploring faith-based resources or incorporating spiritual practices into one's daily routine in order to support mental health recovery.

Community Outreach Programs: Community outreach programs are designed to provide resources and support to members of a community. They can involve offering educational programming, providing financial aid, hosting social events, and more.

Language Barriers: Language barriers refer to challenges in communication due to differences in language or dialects. This includes individuals who do not speak the same native language as well as those with accents that may be difficult for others to understand.

Culturally-Sensitive Services: Culturally-sensitive services are mental health services that are tailored to an individual's unique cultural needs and experiences. These can include providing interpreters for individuals who need assistance communicating, connecting patients with culturally appropriate providers or resources, and understanding how cultural values can affect mental health.

Support Networks: Support networks are groups of individuals who come together to provide emotional or practical support during difficult times. This can involve friends, family members, support groups, religious organizations, and other social networks.

Resilience: Resilience is the ability to recover quickly from adversity or trauma. It involves having a sense of hope and optimism as well as the skills needed to overcome challenges and build on successes.

Stereotypes: Stereotypes are broadly-shared assumptions about the characteristics and behavior of individuals belonging to certain groups. They can be based on race, gender, sexual orientation, religion, culture, socio-economic status, etc., but are often inaccurate or outdated. Stereotypes can lead to prejudice and discrimination and should be challenged whenever possible.

Inclusive Representation: Inclusive representation refers to the accurate and respectful portrayal of individuals from different backgrounds in the media. It involves avoiding stereotypes, presenting a wide range of experiences, and creating content that is both informative and entertaining for audiences.

Access to Care: Access to care refers to the ability of individuals to obtain necessary healthcare services. It can be impacted by factors such as cost, availability of providers, language barriers, stigma, and cultural norms.

Quality Care: Quality care is healthcare that meets or exceeds established standards in terms of effectiveness and safety. This includes timely access to appropriate treatments and services as well as personalized care tailored to an individual's needs.

Additional Resources

The Stigma of Mental Health in the African American Community is a valuable resource for anyone looking to gain knowledge, understanding, and encouragement about seeking help for their mental health struggles. While having access to the information in this book is an important first step in overcoming stigma and getting help, there are several additional resources available that can provide further support on the journey.

Here are some book resources for further reading and learning:

1. *The Black Mental Health Workbook: Break the Stigma, Find Space for Reflection, and Reclaim Self-Care* by Jasmine Lamitte.

2. *The Unapologetic Guide to Black Mental Health: Navigate an Unequal System, Learn Tools for Emotional Wellness, and Get the Help You Deserve* by Dr. Rheeda Walker.

3. *Bipolar Faith: A Black Woman's Journey with Depression and Faith* by Monica A. Coleman.

4. *The Color of Hope: People of Color Mental Health Narratives* by Vanessa Hazzard and M. Nicole Hazzard.

Here are some online communities or forums for Black individuals to discuss mental health:

1. Black Mental Health Community Forum by Family Institute: Offers resources on how to become a Black Men Heal Provider or Clinician, as well as free therapy sessions.

2. Melanin & Mental Health Directory: A comprehensive directory of mental health professionals that specialize in the African American community.

3. Black Girls Breathing: A community for Black women to manage stress through a combination of breathwork techniques.

4. Black Men Heal: An online tool for finding free mental health services specifically geared toward Black men.

These resources are designed to provide further knowledge, support, and assistance when it comes to overcoming the stigma of mental health in the African American community. We hope this book and these resources will help you on your journey to getting the help and support that you need.

Acknowledgments

This book would not have been possible without the help of many people. I am deeply thankful for those in the African American community who shared their stories of mental health stigma with me. Without their bravery and willingness to speak openly about their experiences, this book would not have been possible.

I am also grateful to the mental health professionals and advocates who provided expertise for this book. Their knowledge and dedication to providing quality care to those in need are truly remarkable, and I am thankful for their insight and guidance.

I would like to thank my friends, family, and colleagues who have supported me throughout this project. Your encouragement has been invaluable, and I am truly grateful.

Finally, I want to thank all of the readers who pick up this book and take time to learn more about mental health in the African American community. I hope that it helps provide you with knowledge, understanding, and a sense of comfort as you continue on your journey toward better mental health.

Thank you!

Author's Note

As the author of this book, I feel deeply passionate about raising awareness and destigmatizing mental health in African American communities. Mental illness is a serious issue that affects millions of people every day, and I hope this book serves as a resource to help those who are struggling to find the support they need.

I believe that everyone should have equal access to quality mental health care, that stigma should never be an obstacle to seeking help, and that stories of resilience and recovery should be celebrated. I wrote this book with the goal of providing readers with foundational knowledge and resources about mental health in African American communities, as well as inspiration for continuing on their journey toward better mental wellness.

It is my hope that this book will not only help to reduce the stigma around mental illness among African Americans but also prompt more conversations about the importance of mental health within our culture. I believe that by increasing education, accessibility, and advocacy, we can create a safe and supportive community for everyone.

I invite readers to use this book as a guide, exploring the topics that are relevant to them in order to gain knowledge and understanding of mental health. It is my sincere wish that this book helps bring comfort and clarity on your journey toward better emotional well-being.

Thank you for taking the time to read this book.

Warmly,
Antonio Brigham, MSN-Ed, RN

References

1. Rivera, K. J., Zhang, J. Y., Mohr, D. C., Wescott, A. B., & Pederson, A. B. (2021). A narrative review of mental illness stigma reduction interventions among African Americans in The United States. *Journal of mental health & clinical psychology*, *5*(2), 20.

2. Ward, E., Wiltshire, J. C., Detry, M. A., & Brown, R. L. (2013). African American men and women's attitude toward mental illness, perceptions of stigma, and preferred coping behaviors. *Nursing research*, *62*(3), 185.

3. American Psychiatric Association. (2020). *Addressing Mental Health Stigma in African American and Other Communities of Color.*

4. White, R. (2019). Why mental health care is stigmatized in black communities.

5. Snowden, L. R. (2003). Bias in mental health assessment and intervention: Theory and evidence. *American journal of public health*, *93*(2), 239-243.

6. Ward, E. C., Clark, L. O., & Heidrich, S. (2009). African American women's beliefs, coping behaviors, and barriers to seeking mental health services. *Qualitative health research*, *19*(11), 1589-1601.

7. Watkins, D. C., & Neighbors, H. W. An exploratory study of help-seeking intentions among African American men with depression.

8. Hopkins, P. D., & Shook, N. J. (2017). A review of sociocultural factors that may underlie differences in African American and European American anxiety. *Journal of Anxiety Disorders*, *49*, 104-113.

9. Ibrahimi, S., Yusuf, K. K., Dongarwar, D., Maiyegun, S. O., Ikedionwu, C., & Salihu, H. M. (2020). COVID-19 devastation of African American families: Impact on mental health and the consequence of systemic racism. *International Journal of Maternal and Child Health and AIDS*, *9*(3), 390.

10. Monk Jr, E. P. (2020). Linked fate and mental health among African Americans. *Social Science & Medicine*, *266*, 113340.

www.ingramcontent.com/pod-product-compliance
Lightning Source LLC
Chambersburg PA
CBHW070044040426
42333CB00041B/2307